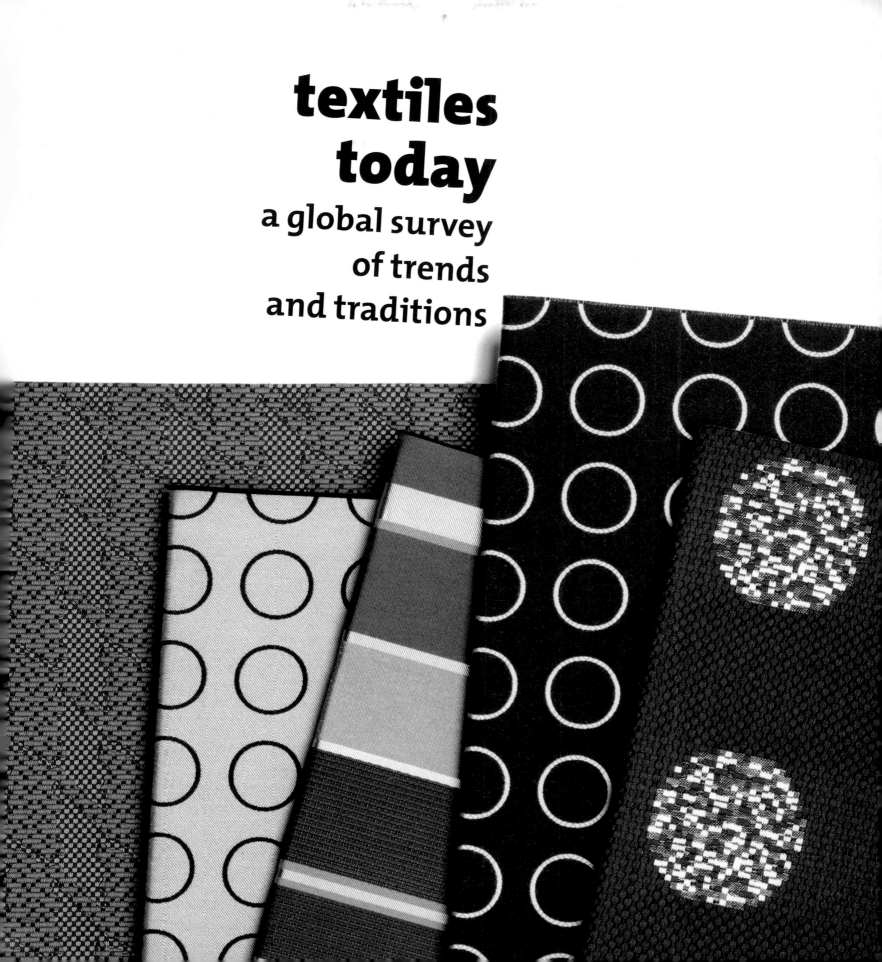

textiles today
a global survey of trends and traditions

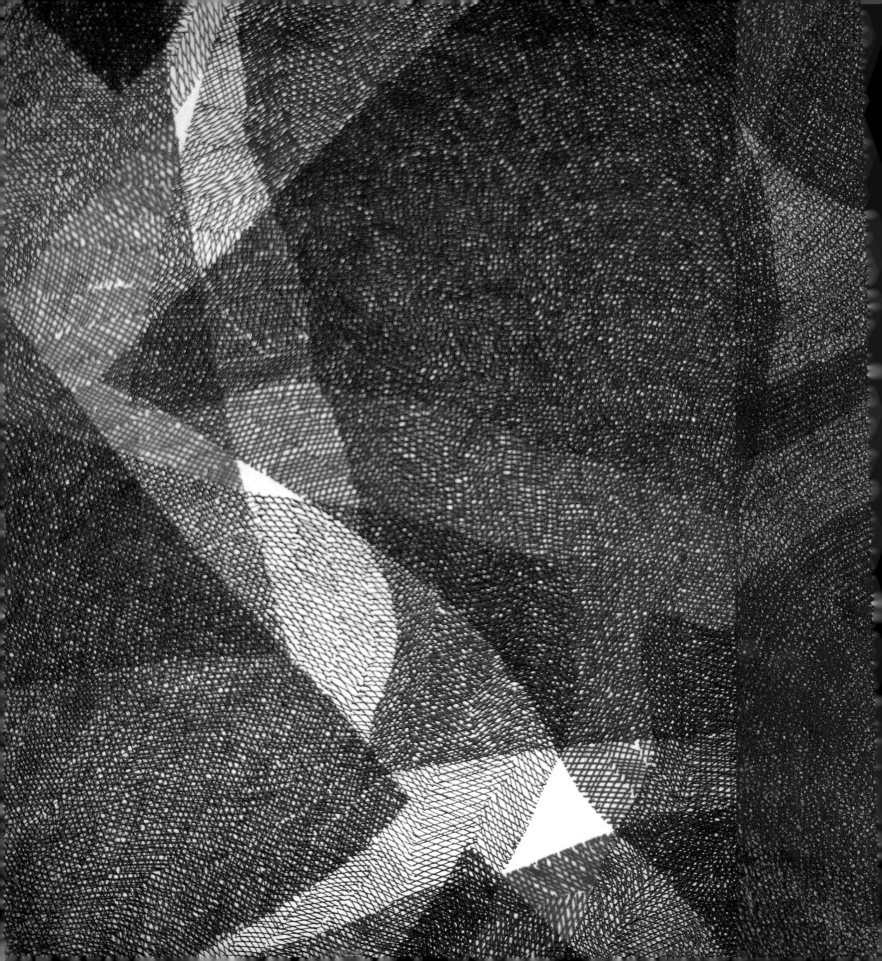

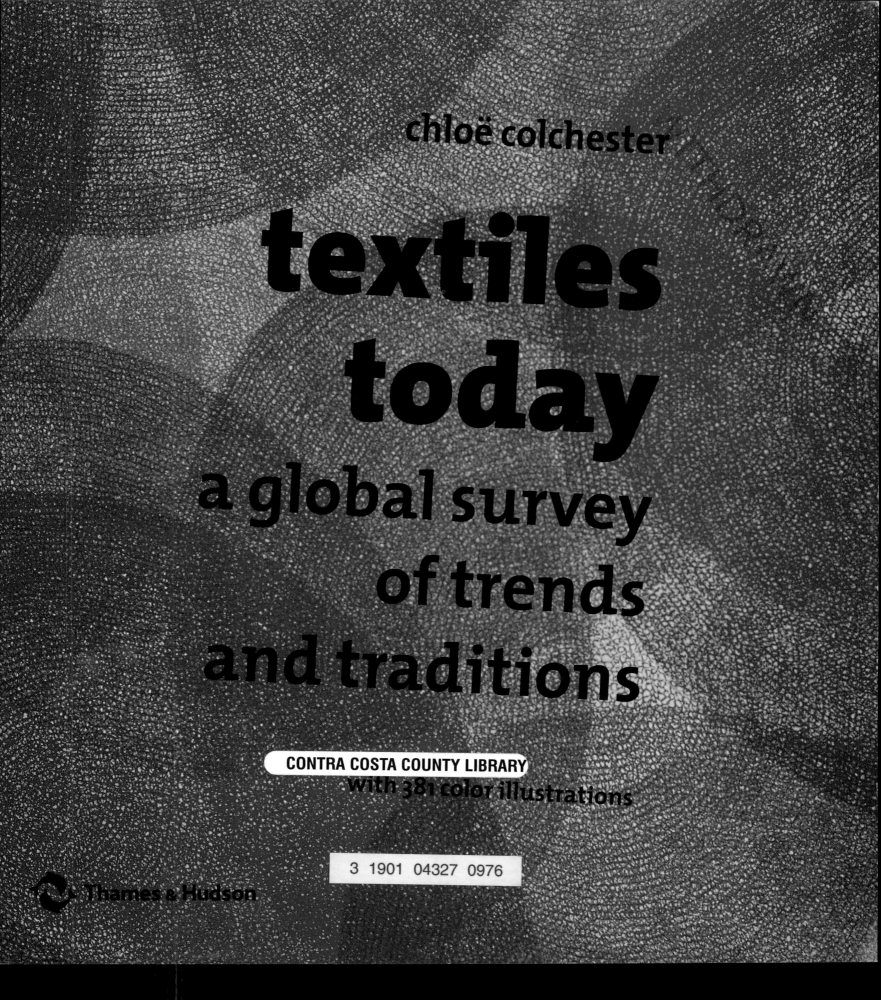

chloë colchester

textiles today

a global survey of trends and traditions

with 381 color illustrations

Thames & Hudson

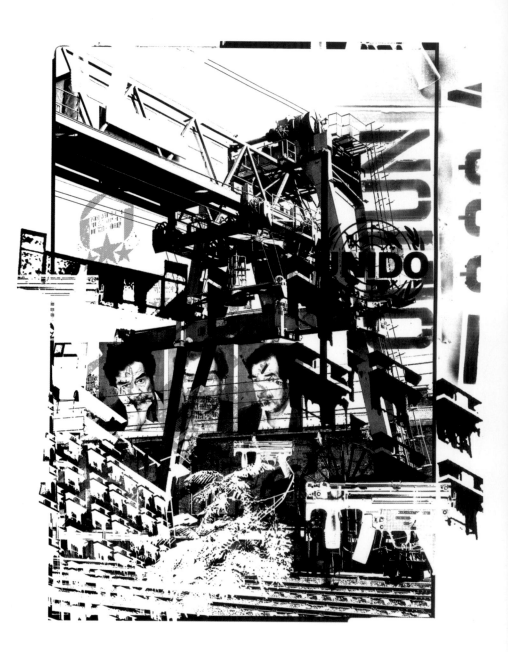

page 1: Hella Jongerius, *Repeat*, Maharam, New York, 2002
pages 2–3: Aurora Caresi, wool felt, 2004
page 4: Nuflo T-shirt design, 2004
page 5: Paola Lenti, *Crochet Rug*, 2004

First published in 2007 in hardcover in the United States
of America by Thames & Hudson Inc., 500 Fifth Avenue,
New York, New York 10110

thamesandhudsonusa.com

Library of Congress Catalog Card Number 2007922780

ISBN 978-0-500-51381-1

Printed in China by Midas Printing International Ltd

contents

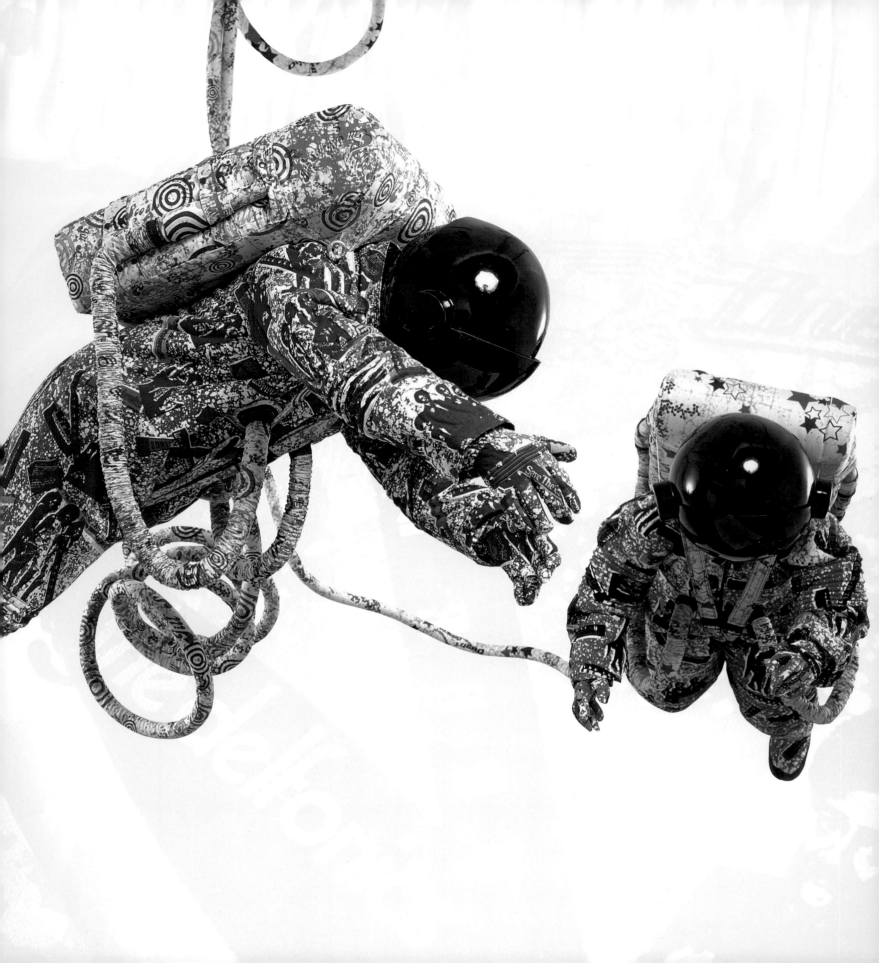

Introduction: Textiles for the 21st Century, a World Wide Survey

Aspects of Innovation

The beginning of the 21st century has witnessed an exceptional period of change and innovation in the science, design and art of textiles. These innovations have two different aspects. On the one hand, they involve materials and prototypes that are so new that we can hardly foresee how the familiar functions of textiles will be transformed in the future: fabrics that can harvest solar energy and emit light or heat, interactive digital textile displays, fabrics that are touch-sensitive, primed to detect a faltering pulse or environmental pollutants, fabric buildings and fabric armour that can change colour, or flex textile muscles, all show how textiles are being fundamentally reinvented for predicted demands in the century ahead of us. But there is also another side of innovation that involves responding intelligently to the textiles with which we live, an approach that can involve addressing some of the consequences and environmental impacts of more than two centuries of industrial innovation and international trade. Thus inevitably our relationship with textiles today is not exclusively forward looking, but means looking sideways, to other parts of the world, and also behind us to the legacy of the import and export of ideas, patterns, fabrics and garment types over time.

Yinka Shonibare (UK), *Spacewalk*, 2002, was commissioned by the Fabric Workshop in Philadelphia, an organization that promotes the use of textiles in art. For this piece, the workshop collaborated with the artist to produce a range of screen prints. The patterns draw upon Philadelphia soul album covers and the tradition of African wax prints.

Surveying contemporrary textiles from around the world today reveals a field that is very diverse; this diversity is both exciting and provocative because it involves bringing together a range of otherwise fragmented images and perspectives of the future. This is challenging because the future is often viewed through a telescope that focuses upon developments in science and technology to the exclusion of everything else, for instance, the cultural dimensions of our lives. The resurgence of technology-led visions of the future at the turn of the millennium was – and remains – understandable given the excitement of the introduction of e-textiles (the cross over between communications technology and textiles) and other developments in the material science of textiles promised by nanotechnology (a field of material design where components are of an equivalent scale to atoms and molecules in the natural world). But textiles are a fundamental part of our every daily lives and their development can never be solely attributed to technology. Like music or food, textiles are at once one of the most and least localized of the arts: they owe their development to religion, commerce, cultural exchange and travel, and their preservation to tenacious regionalism. It is these dynamics that make people not only care for textiles, but also care intimately *about* them, while simultaneously connecting them to the forces at work in the broader economy.

Contemporary fashion and interior fabrics are propelled by the aesthetics of cultural transfer: vintage clothes, work wear, 19th-century prints, patterns long since derived and adapted from Asian originals meet together in looping analogies and new combinations. Cultural exchange was a major catalyst for the Industrial Revolution in the 18th century. In the 16th century Europeans were dazzled by the beauty and technical sophistication of textile goods that had emerged as a result of over four centuries inter-Asian trade. As early as the 17th century both Chinese and Indian garments began to be worn by European men and in the 18th century the influx of chintzes, Indian block-printed fabrics and later Kashmir shawls, each subtly adapted to appeal to European women, led to the mechanization of weaving, and subsequently to the development of the jacquard loom – innovations that helped to tip control of the world trade to the West by paving the way for the mechanization of other industries and eventually, in the second half of the 20th century, for the emergence of the digital age.

We are all familiar with the account of technological development that leads, via a discussion of international modernism and the aspirations of the space age, to the information society of the present day. If we are less accustomed to viewing the same subject in a different light and on a broader historical scale – by following a thread through the

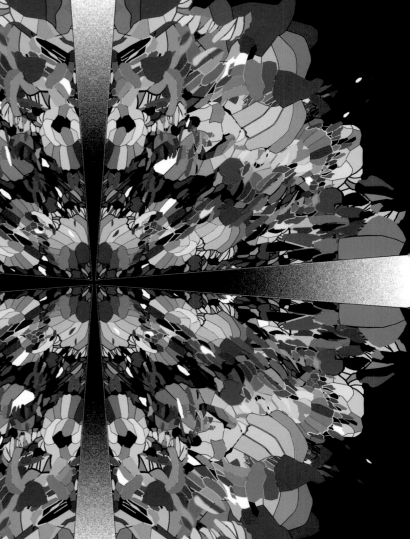

Jonathan Saunders(UK), *Bauhaus Rose*,
Summer 2005.

Manish Arora (India), Hand-embroidered
dress entitled *Love*, from the Winter
2006/2007 collection.

slave cotton plantations to the American civil rights movement of the 1960s, or through the export of cheap manufactured cottons to captive colonial markets in India, Africa and the East Indies to the resurgence of textiles as a medium of post-colonial cultural expression in art and fashion today – it may be because museum displays of traditional textiles from other cultures have blinded us to the broader consequences of textile commerce and industrial development for so long.

That particular excuse no longer exists. For the past two decades contemporary artists and designers of international standing, from Africa and the Pacific, have drawn upon indigenous textile traditions and colonial textiles, or the hybrid fabrics that have developed from cultural exchange over time, as a means of investigating art culture and politics in the colonial and post-colonial epochs. Fabrics have also figured prominently in work concerning the relationship between First Nation peoples and settler communities in different parts of the New World. More recently, British and French artists and designers from different ethnic backgrounds, such as India, Mali, Madagascar, Morocco, Burkina Faso and Nigeria, have reinvigorated art and fashion by using the colonial fabrics and graphic elements they find on the streets of Paris and London to project an alternative, synoptic vision of textile culture on the international stage. These significant initiatives have inspired museums and academics to adjust their perspective accordingly. It is important to the work of many of these artists and designers that cloth is patterned. In their hands patterned cloth has become a device for seeing the world, for conveying the vast dimensions, often tragic, often governed by mutual misunderstanding, of human destiny on the wider scale. Their work could therefore not be more different from the hidebound parochialism that was (very often wrongly) imputed to indigenous textile traditions. Yet, since pattern is used as a way of exploring a relationship, the provenance of a piece of work becomes difficult to pin down. Accordingly, the book is organized thematically as opposed to regionally.

Interactive and dynamic patterns are also a feature of e-textiles. By combining thermo-chromic inks (which change colour at different temperatures) with conductive fibres and a heat element patterns can be made to shift and change in response to an external electronic signal. As yet, research into clothing equipped to communicate through interactive digital displays of pattern and graphics remains in early stages of development, yet experimental designers have played a key role by working with the limited materials available to reveal the potential of this field. Partly as a result of their efforts research into fibres with enhanced optical properties has now started to develop in earnest. This

Ronan and Erwan Bouroullec (France), *North Tiles*, 2006. The installation of textile tiles in Kvadrat's showroom was inspired by the scales of a fish. The design is modular and adaptable. Each tile is composed of a solid foam core which is sandwiched between two layers of cloth. The partitions are easy to assemble and disassemble and can be adapted to form different enclosures.

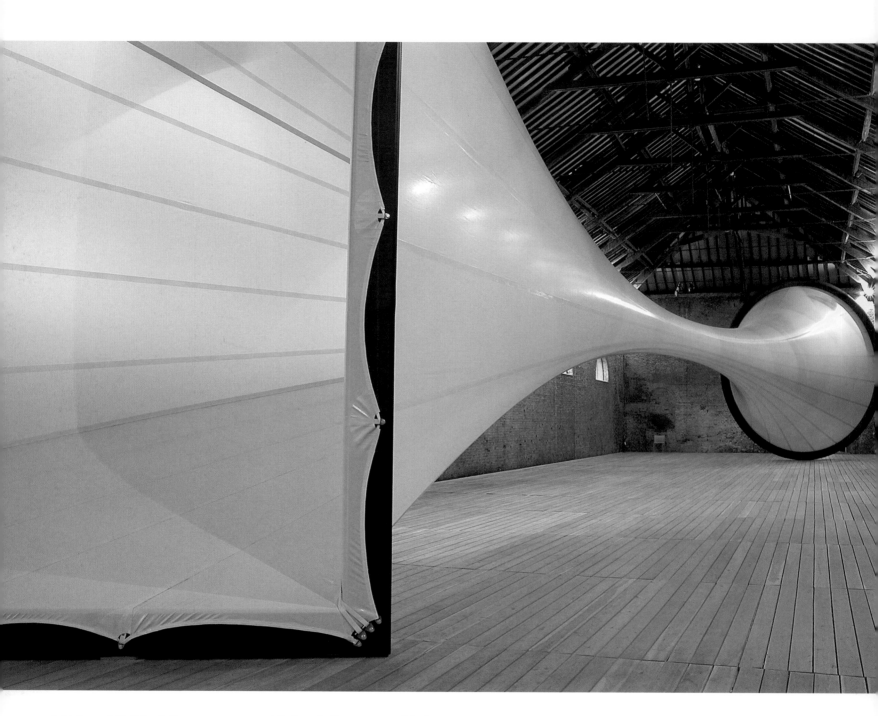

Anish Kapoor (UK), *Melancholia*, 2004.
A pvc-coated textile by Hightex that draws
upon research by Arup Associates for the
Marsayas project. The geometry of tensile
membrane structures is based on the
behaviour of soap bubble forms. Arup

used the form-finding programme Fabwin
to simulate the behaviour of soap films.
These basic geometric forms were stretched
and adapted until the right degree of
attenuation was achieved.

12

implies a great shift. Material scientists have tended to limit their attention to the physical characteristics of materials – their strength, porosity, resilience and so on; now, following Japan's lead, they are beginning to develop fibres with enhanced optical, acoustic and olfactory properties.

These developments have attracted the interest of experimental product designers who have used new fabrics to create a range of objects, buildings and experimental shelters. However questions about the nature of creativity raised by chaos theory and post-modernism have also prompted a marked revival of interest in pattern in the work of avant-garde Dutch and Scandinavian product designers. Computer modelling (especially parallel processing) has generated interest in spontaneous processes of pattern formation that are characteristic of complex, distributed systems formed by a large number of similar units that are governed by simple rules of interaction. At the same time, the more responsive approach to creativity ushered in by post-modernism has, among other concerns, provoked an interest in genre, dressing up and has, with pre-modern vernacular folk art traditions, also contributed to a revival of interest in patterned fabric as a vehicle for cultural transmission. Because internet relay chat is helping to restore the collaborative dimension of art activity it may even contribute to the development of new traditions of folk art.

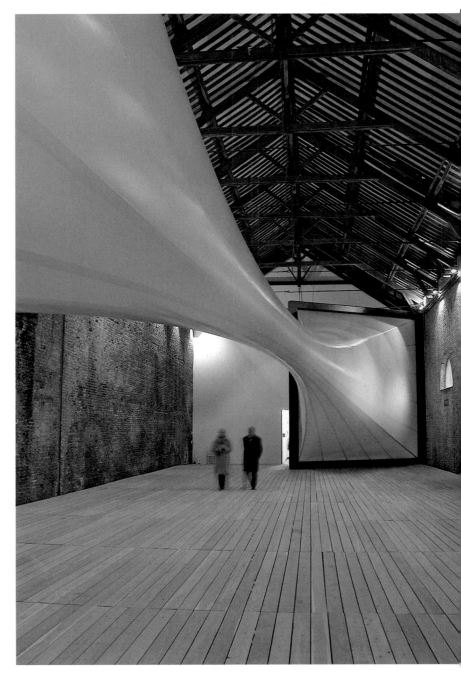

Protected Innovation

Changing attitudes to top-down, inside-out design may be legitimated by intellectual movements, but they are also a feature of the rise of consumer culture. The 1980s and 1990s witnessed a decisive change of attitude towards textile and fashion design as the power of high street retailers increased. Rather than fashion being defined by designers from Paris, Milan and New York, whose clothes could only be afforded by the rich, retailers began to experiment with different lines and styles to see what was palatable through digital marketing, which allowed designs to be tried and tested in the market place. More important still, digital communication allowed amazingly cheap fashion to be mass-marketed by enabling retailers to maintain control of the design while out sourcing textile and garment manufacture to low-wage countries. Initially heralded as a breakthrough for consumer choice, it is only a decade on, now that high streets and shopping malls have become increasingly homogenized in Britain and the United States that, owing to concerns about the cultural and environmental impacts of globalization, we have started to question the parameters of our choice.

Yet by the mid-1990s the gradual shift from a production to a demand-led economy had strengthened the case for reforming the age-old system of trade restrictions that had previously protected textile production in the West. Initially, developing countries were encouraged to open up their markets to overseas competition; then it was the turn of the richer countries. January, 2005 was to have marked the culmination of a ten-year programme where one major plank of European and American trade defences – the existing regime of quotas – was lifted.

The protection of Europe and America's textile industry, along with agriculture, had long been seen as one of the great anomalies within GATT (the General Agreements on Tariffs and Trade), the third pillar, along with the World Bank and the International Monetary Fund, of the international trading system that was established in the aftermath of the Second World War. Despite repeated calls for market liberalization the textile industry had remained protected by import duties (tariffs), quotas (which limit the quantity of specific categories of textiles and clothing goods that can be exported by developing countries to richer nations) and farming subsidies.

The system of quotas began as 'temporary' trade limits intended to stem the flood of Japanese cottons to the West in the 1950s. By the end of the decade quotas had been extended to other countries such as India, Pakistan and Hong Kong where low labour costs also made their products dangerously competitive. Then in the 1960s quotas were imposed to stem the surge of textiles from rapidly developing industrial economies such as China, South Korea, Bangladesh, Vietnam,

Cambodia and Sri Lanka into developed industrial economies such as the European Union, Canada, Finland, Norway and the United States.

For advocates of free trade, unfolding and extending the industrial revolution to other parts of the world and lifting barriers to export was seen as the best path to raising standards of living and eradicating global poverty. According to their view, trade restrictions were perceived as an iniquitous barrier to developing countries and an anachronism in terms of contemporary trade.

However, the progressive liberalization of Euro-American textile markets at the turn of the millennium coincided with the emergence of China as a major manufacturing base for textiles, clothing, toys and electronic goods. Its accession to the World Trade Organization in 2001 also ensured it a prominent place in multilateral trade negotiations. While major textile companies such as Burlington, Courtaulds, Coats Viyella and ICI fabrics closed their doors, the press began documenting stories of factories along the Pearl River Delta employing thousands of Chinese girls working seven days a week to produce garments for retail chains Zara, a Spanish company, and the Swedish retailer H and M. It was perhaps due to this situation that almost 90 per cent of the quotas of the most price-sensitive categories such as bras, sheets and cheap knitwear were phased out abruptly at the end of the ten-year period.

Within the first few months after these final trade restrictions were lifted in January, 2005 China's exports of clothing to Europe surged by 45 per cent, plunging the European textile industry into one of the worst trade disputes in its history. Between April and August, 75–80 million Chinese-produced bras, T-shirts, jumpers and other items of clothing piled up in bonded warehouses along Europe's borders, prompting quotas to be reimposed on certain categories of garments exported from China.

In Europe the row over quotas revealed a split in trade between the luxury markets and clothing markets. The split marked a divide between street retailers in Denmark, Finland, Germany, the Netherlands, Sweden and Britain, who, since the 1980s, have sourced clothing from all over the world and tend to be in favour of market liberalization, and clothing producers in France, Italy, Spain, Portugal (half of the 2 million EU textile and clothing jobs are in the last three), the Czech Republic, Poland and Slovakia, who are in favour of maintaining quota restrictions and rules of origin. From an international perspective the crisis has confirmed fears that China and India are likely to benefit most from the liberalization. The World Trade Organization predicts that China will soon control 50 per cent of the world's textile trade. This means that other smaller, more vulnerable economies such as

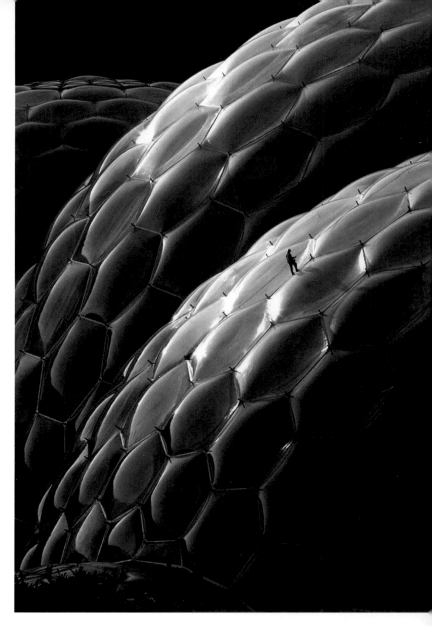

Cambodia, Bangladesh and Sri Lanka, who rely on textiles and clothing for the vast majority of their exports, or countries that have had preferential access to American and European markets could see their industries suffer seriously as result of market reform.

Euro-American dominance of textile production and design, which has remained constant for the past two centuries, is also beginning to falter. It is over twenty years since the international design community became aware of the work of the Japanese textile designers of genius, for instance, Junichi Arai and Rai Kawakubo, who began reworking craft traditions such as those of Kiryu, a weaving centre, through the use of new materials, polyester and springy over-spun cotton computerized weaving and experimental heat treatment and finishes. In the intervening period South Korea and Taiwan have begun to produce technology-rich fabrics of note and India has begun to develop a fashion industry that is every bit as international as that of Japan.

China, which has invested in a five-year plan to restructure its textile and clothing industries and to develop technology-rich synthetics, may soon follow suit. It now wants to make its own clothing brands rather than being the manufacturing arm of Europe and has begun outsourcing its production to countries such as Bangladesh. These developments have prompted some observers to draw an analogy between the current resurgence of design in China and India and the former pre-eminence of these countries in inter-Asian exchange prior to the 18th century. They suggest that the topography of the global economy has begun to re-orient itself and the century ahead will be marked by a shift from a world governed by a 'single peak' to a far more varied terrain marked by the re-emergence of capitals of design and consumption in the Far East.

Eden Project (2001), Cornwall, ETFE-coated membrane by Vector Foiltec (UK/Germany).

The Revival of Modernism
in the 21st century

The revival of belief in modernist values, in science, technology and production-led innovation, occurred within the context of market liberalization inspired by the development of consumer culture. It was expressed in the use of state-of-the-art fabrics for major public building projects, such as the Millennium Dome (1999) and the Eden Project (2001), two British buildings that were intended to present a dynamic, forward-looking vision of the future through re-invoking early 20th-century modernist precedents. More recently, vast membrane structures, such as the 70,000 seater Allianz Arena football stadium in Munich (2005) and the forthcoming National Swimming Centre, known as the Water Cube, for the 2008 Beijing Olympics, designed by the Australian architects P⁻W, have reworked the modernist idiom of youthful fitness, health and exercise as a metaphor for a bright future in a different, 21st-century setting. We are also witnessing the revival of the early modernists' utopian vision of the potential of new technology to create a better world. Design is becoming more humanitarian. State-of-the-art technologies may allow the rich nations to redress the balance by providing shelter, light and power supplies to assist refugees or people living in remote communities.

Smart materials are no longer passive and inert but responsive; some are even active. They respond to external stimulae: to heat, to light, to pressure and to chemical changes; and they can act by changing shape, or harvesting solar energy, or conducting electricity and light, or by conveying sensory data; or transmitting light in the way that natural materials, sometimes pejoratively referred to as 'dumb materials', cannot. Many of these materials are the result of efforts to combine textile technology with plastic electronics and information technology (IT) which took place in the 1990s.

It is above all, the recent developments in nanotechnology that have prompted speculation that we may be embarking on a new technological revolution, every bit as significant as the Industrial Revolution in the 18th century, involving the redesign of materials on the atomic scale. Ever since IBM rearranged 35 xenon atoms with a scanning tunnelling microscope to spell out the letters of its corporate logo in 1989, it has been widely accepted that we can manipulate matter at the atomic scale.

Textiles have been some of the first products to be marketed on the basis of their nanoscale finishes. It should perhaps be pointed out that most of these fabrics incorporate catalysts or precision manufacturing techniques used in the manufacture of semi-conductors and fibre optics that were developed long before the massive investment in nanotechnology took place. Research into molecular manufacture

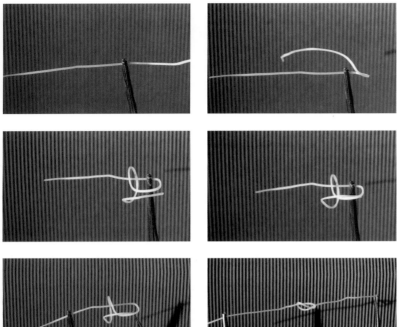
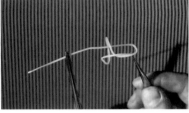
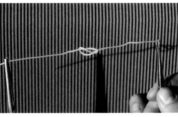

Andreas Lendlein (mNemoscience, Germany), 2002. Sequence of images showing the world's first 'intelligent' suture tying itself into a knot within 20 seconds when it is exposed to 41 degrees centigrade. In 1997, while working at MIT, Lendlein developed a shape memory polymer that would respond to body temperature. Shape memory materials can memorize a permanent shape and are automatically transformed into this permanent shape when exposed to a suitable external trigger such as body heat. Lendlein's sutures are designed for keyhole surgery and are made from polymeric material that encourages tissue renewal and biodegrade naturally within the body. The sutures are now being developed for commercial production. mNemoscience is currently working on light-sensitive shape memory materials.

still remains at a very early stage. Scientists are divided as to whether it will be possible to scale down versions of the gears, rotors and bearings used in conventional engineering at the atomic or molecular level, or promote more forms of self-assembly, or whether to develop materials through a closer study of the way that biological materials are developed in the natural world and computer-assisted chemical engineering.

At the moment atomic probes only afford us a static picture of the surface of natural materials, but research scientists have already begun to envisage the next stage when they will enable us to develop a more dynamic view of how natural materials respond to external stimulae. Far from natural materials appearing dumb, it would seem that we are only just beginning to realize what they may be able to teach us.

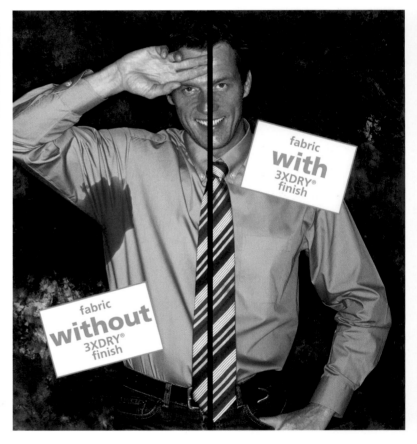

3xdry manufactured by Schoeller Textil AG was developed in conjunction with Ciba Speciality Chemicals AG in 2001. The shirt was designed to overcome sweat-soaked armpits, a problem with poly-cotton shirts. The cloth is finished in such a way that it displays both hydrophilic (moisture absorbing) and hydrophobic (water-repellent) properties. The material allows sweat to wick away from the body comfortably and invisibly.

The Industrial Context

The current generation of new materials emerging from industrially developed nations in Europe and from the United States, Japan and South Korea surveyed here represent material scientists' most dazzling attempts yet to create highly specialized and technically complex materials that will enable them to outperform the increasingly sophisticated synthetics from other parts of the world. Yet the industrial context is markedly varied in different parts of the world.

Japan and South Korea still retain a critical mass of chemical companies and fibre manufacturers such as Mitsubushi, Teijin, Toyobo and Hyosung who continue to lead research in the field. Here the approach to research remains secretive and relatively closed to public enquiries. In Europe and the United States, the closure of synthetic giants, such as Courtaulds and Burlington, means that research is now increasingly in the hands of academic scientists, working independently from the established textile industry; many of whom start up their own businesses to manufacture their inventions. Outsourcing research to independent academics has even become a feature of defence research.

Heavy investment in military technology has been a defining feature of the American economy since the Great Depression in the 1930s – sufficient time for a military-led model of technological innovation to become deeply embedded in its culture. What is called the NASA effect is the process whereby significant innovations developed for the military or aerospace industries are then re-adapted for civilian use: nylon, T-Shirts, Goretex and the Internet are renowned examples and have all had an impact upon the textile industry today. Yet changing circumstances – the cost of the war in Iraq and the changing nature of warfare – have begun to put pressure on the budgets for new weapons. Although defence spending on new weapon systems, which fell to $50 billion after the collapse of the Berlin Wall, were revived to Cold War levels under the first Bush Administration (1989–93), the scale of the defence budget has once again started to be challenged. Orders for massively expensive military hardware such as the stealth fighter and the new joint striker, naval destroyers and aircraft carriers are declining.

Now increasing attention is focused on the Pentagon's second largest defence programme, Future Combat Systems, a $165 billion project to upgrade the Army's vehicles, communication systems and uniforms. One arm of this, the Future Force Warrior Programme, aims to create technologically enhanced military uniforms with the intention of making individual soldiers more capable and responsive in situations of urban guerrilla conflict by giving them access to battlefield information from satellites and unmanned aircraft.

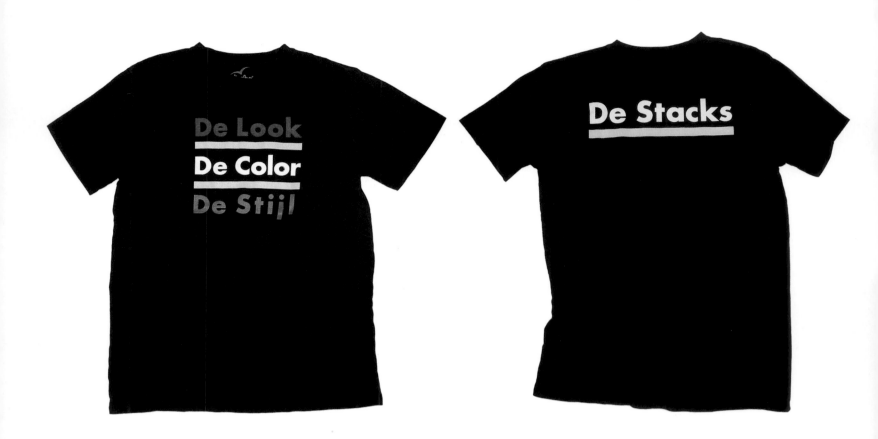

The interesting thing is how much of the Future Force Warrior Programme is open to public scrutiny. For example, the Institute for Soldier Nanotechnologies at MIT (the Massachusetts Institute for Technology) set up in 2002 was given $50 million from the American Defence Budget and a further $50 million from private sponsors such as DuPont. The university's commitment to the open dissemination of knowledge means that it will not undertake classified research. Instead, it has provided detailed progress reports of its research to the media, who eagerly monitor the marvellous fabrics it is working on: for instance, uniforms equipped with textile muscles that can boost a soldier's muscle capacity fivefold; ferromagnetic fabric uniforms that can suddenly stiffen into armour; spider silk combat gear; colour-changing, light-sensitive camouflage.

Will the NASA effect work in this case? Will these specialist, highly engineered fabrics give popular culture its distinctive physical expression as mass-produced clothing and mass-produced synthetics – nylon, polyester, lycra, cellulose – did in the second half of the 20th century? Some people believe such fabrics will remain relegated to specialist niche markets of ski-wear, protective apparel and health vests designed to monitor the elderly and will leave the fashion, interiors and technical textile markets broadly unchanged. Others believe that the smart textiles and nanotechnology are part of a much bigger revolution in material design that will, according to Janine Benyus, effect a 'transition from an industrial system organised on the basis of the idea that material is cheap and that shape is expensive…to one where material is expensive and the shape is comparatively cheap.'

Commonwealth Stacks was launched from an apartment in Los Angeles in 2000 by Laura and Michael Leon. They use T-shirts as a platform for thoughtful design.

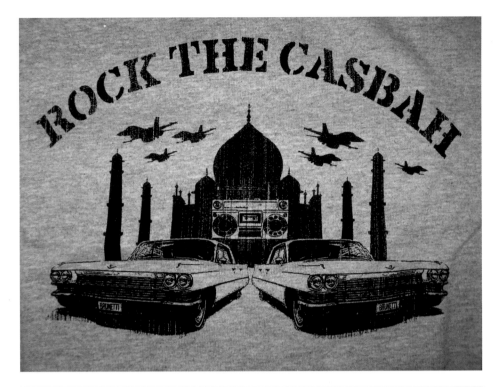

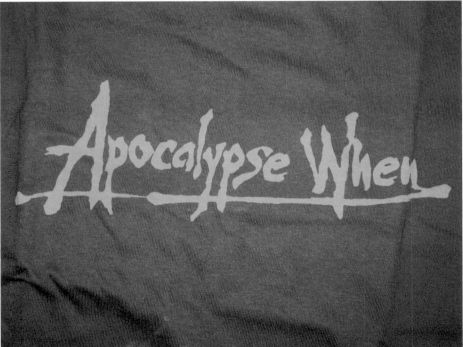

Fuct is a clothing brand started by graffiti
artist and writer Eric Brunetti from Venice
Beach, California, in 1991.

The Cost of Materials and the Global Economy

Growing consciousness of the world's limits, of dwindling fossil fuels and raw materials have made us question the world view of the first phase of industrial manufacture that saw materials as cheap and endlessly renewable and fashion as a primary stimulant to demand. There is now a growing awareness that we need to change the way that we have been living our lives, the way we shop, the amount we consume, the chemicals and materials involved in textile production and fabric care, what we do with waste clothing – all need to alter. At the industrial level, concerns that the textile and clothing supply systems created through global sourcing are becoming unsustainable in terms of environmental impact are leading many people to the conclusion that the textile and clothing industry needs to be entirely rethought to meet the demands ahead of us.

Because the textile and clothing industries have become deeply economically and culturally entrenched in a particular way of doing things this transformation implies not simply a new technological solution, but also a profound cultural transformation. Design is important here because it can help to bring about a shift in the collective imagination. There are now a growing number of internet sites and eco-design portals that promote and discuss the work by experimental designers who have begun to move towards sustainable consumption by creating multifunctional objects or who refashion high-value products from second-hand clothing, used truck tarpaulins, plastic bags and other forms of waste. While some of these designs are sustainable only in the restricted sense that they use second-hand materials, they are helping to transfer concerns that used to belong to the ecological fringe into mainstream thinking. Products that promote the fact that they are energy harvesting are also a move in the right direction. Yet much more needs to be done to convince rich consumers that they can learn to

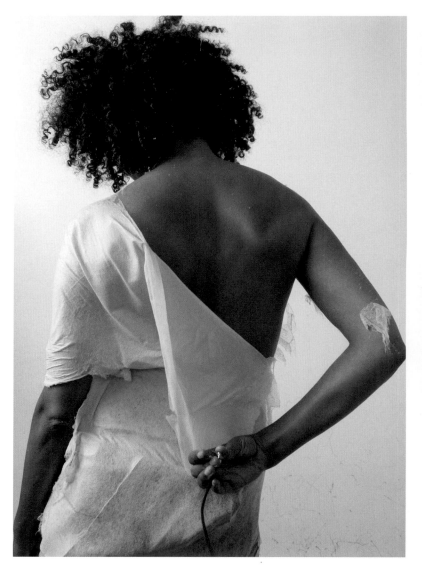

Manel Torres (Spain), FabriCan is a spray-on, non-woven fabric. It consists of fibres and a binder; users can control the thickness of the fabrics they want to achieve by using the spray can in a particular manner. Torres developed the fabric for his doctoral research at the Royal College of Art, London, and he is now developing the material at Imperial College, London.

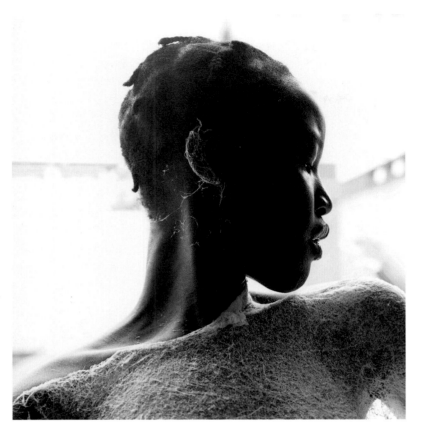

live with less. And at a more profound level ecological design requires addressing what textiles are made from and the way in which they are manufactured and produced.

Both the advent of new textile technologies and new concerns about sustainability present immense challenges for the design profession and for textile design education more generally. The old division between material science training for textile technologists and a grounding in the applied arts for art school courses in textile design is no longer adequate to meet the demands ahead. Just as material scientists are becoming material designers, textile designers will need to revalue the vocational aspects of their training that deal with the detailed aspects of textile manufacture and production and to develop the kind of know-how that will enable them to respond intelligently to new materials and new technologies in the years to come.

At a third level, sustainable design involves changing our relationship to the global market. At present disposable consumption is deeply embedded in our culture and is one of the dynamos of demand which drives the economy. Every year European consumers discard 5.8 million tons of textiles of which, 1.5 million tons are recycled locally through charity shops, 1 million tons exported to the developing world, 50,000 tons recycled into rags, while the other two thirds is burnt or put into landfill. Environmental concerns have meant that consumers have begun to question the relationship between the price of the goods they buy and their cost to the environment.

Although the price of garments may be falling, in the era of increased trade due to global sourcing the environmental impacts caused by agriculture and intensive transportation are increasing. In this respect, cotton is by no means the most natural choice. Cotton remains the principal raw material of the world's textile industry and, despite the fact that many varieties of cotton exist, years of intensive monoculture have made it the most pesticide-intensive crop on the market.

According to the Organic Trade Association, a 1/3 of a pound of agricultural chemicals is used to produce a single cotton T-shirt. Although only 2.4 per cent of the world's arable land is planted with cotton it accounts for a quarter of the global pesticide market and 11 per cent of the insecticide market. Cotton agriculture pollutes ground-water systems and leaves poisonous residues in the milk and meat of the cattle that feed off cottonseed and contaminates food made from cottonseed oil.

Today, 11 million growers raise cotton in the West African countries of Benin, Burkina Faso, Chad, Côte d'Ivoire, Mali and Senegal for the international market. In a vicious twist of history, these millions of African farmers are undercut by merely 35,000 or so mainly white farmers working in the former slave states of Texas and the American south. Nearly $4 billion a year of American federal subsidies allows the United States to produce enough cotton for 9 billion T-shirts to be put on the international market, depressing the market price. In May, 2006 prices for cotton fell to their lowest point since the Great Depression in the 1930s.

A landmark World Trade Organization ruling in 2005 decided that much of the assistance broke their rules of fair trade. In February, 2006 the US senate and house of representatives scrapped the explicit cotton subsidy, yet hand outs for farmers were soon reintegrated under another, more general subsidy scheme that compensates farmers for low commodity prices. The United States now says that it is not prepared to agree to cuts in cotton independently from an overall deal

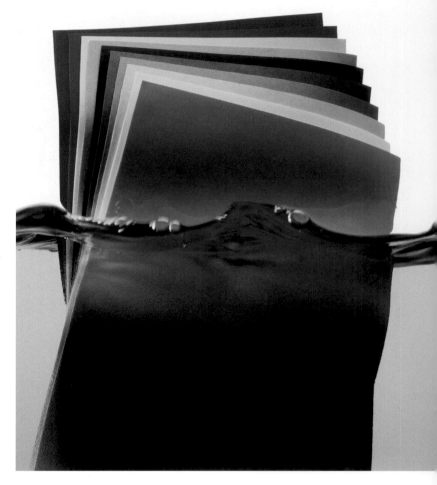

on agriculture – an impasse that is characteristic of the way that slow-moving multi-lateral trade talks tend to develop.

The fairtrade accreditation scheme in the Netherlands in 1988 has recently extended from food into cotton T-shirts, a move that has been much publicised in Britain (still the most enthusiastic supporter for this movement, with the Netherlands and Germany and to a lesser extent Japan following behind) where a new brand of celebrity-endorsed cotton T-shirts has been introduced on the high street. In this new initiative, small co-operatives from Mali and Senegal are guaranteed a return for their crop above the market price which insulates them

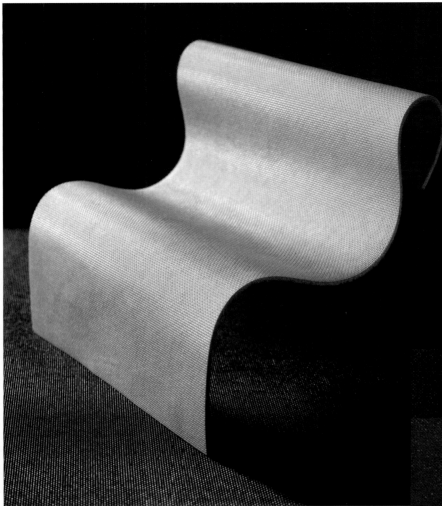

Waterborn is a new synthetic fibre upholstery fabric manufactured almost entirely without the use of organic solvents. It was developed by Kvadrat in close co-operation with a leading fibre producer in Japan. Organic solvents were avoided by using polyurethane dispersed in water to impregnate a non-woven fabric made of polyester and nylon. By heating the fabric, the polyurethane covers the fibres, creating a composite fabric. As a result, organic solvent emissions are reduced to approximately 8 per cent of conventional production emissions. The surface qualities of Waterborn were designed by French architect Jean Nouvel.

against other artificial distortions of the international market. It is a small gesture, perhaps, and one that is hardly likely to change the world trading system fundamentally, even though it may help marginalized producers, but it is another indication that textiles are being viewed in a new way.

Textiles for the Future

Textiles have always been analysed from different perspectives, involving various levels of abstraction and detail: the macro-scale models used by classical economists to analyse global trade abstract fabric to numbers, quality to price; at another level, there exists the particularizing vision, found in books, shops, museums and magazines, where broader considerations can often get lost in the fascination with surface qualities of particular fabrics; beneath this, the synthetics industry has also made us aware of another level of abstraction, the mystifying models of molecular structure developed by chemists.

If these questions of perspective seem more important today than ever before it may be because we are becoming aware of the limitations of this squint-eyed view of the world, uneasily skewed between particularity and abstraction. Atomic-scale probes, for example, are transforming material science by showing us the surface qualities of materials at the atomic and molecular level. More important still, our particularizing vision of fabric has started to open up. Artists and designers have begun to use pattern and textile design to create a view of the world that is both localized and sensitive to the ramifications of international trade. Young families' self-interested concerns about organic food and the effect of pesticides on their children have begun to move into broader concerns about environmental sustainability and

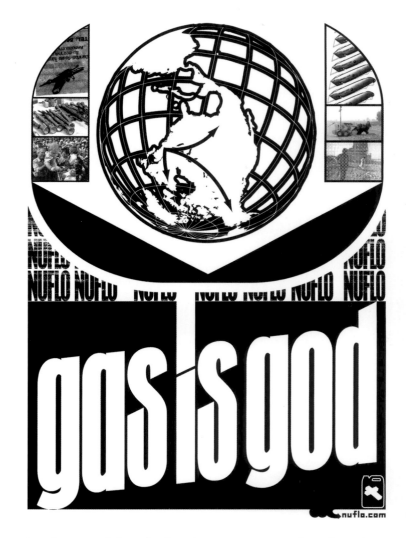

cultural sustainability. The fact that a growing number of people want to know exactly what they are wearing or eating is making designers transform their practice by looking beyond the surface qualities of fabric to the material and energy flows involved in the production and recycling of a piece of cloth. The fairtrade movement is an indication that a growing number of consumers want to look beyond a T-shirt or a piece of cloth to connect directly with the producers.

For William McDonough, an American architect and designer committed to sustainable development, finding an answer to green

Nuflo is a Los Angeles-based independent clothing label founded in 1999.

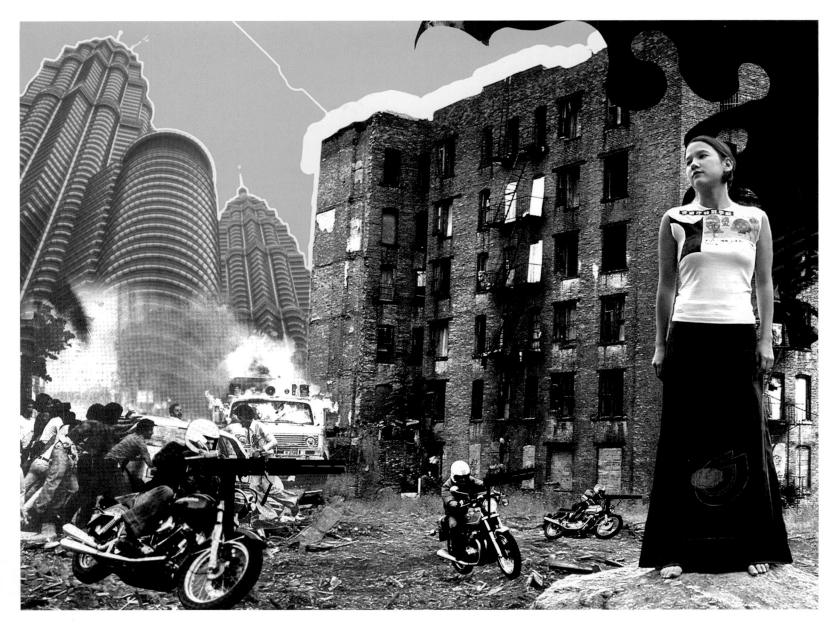

consumption involves a change of attitude that is simultaneously cultural as well as technological. For European and American children raised during the Cold War the threat of nuclear attack and the sense that Armageddon might be imminent encouraged them to have a 'get it while you can' attitude to consumption, a way of living without concern for the morrow. In the aftermath of the Cold War, now that the continuous prosperity of the planet and its ecology has become the primary issue, our perspectives of the future have started to open up. What does our clothing protect us against? What do we want textiles to shelter us from? These are questions that seem more important than ever now.

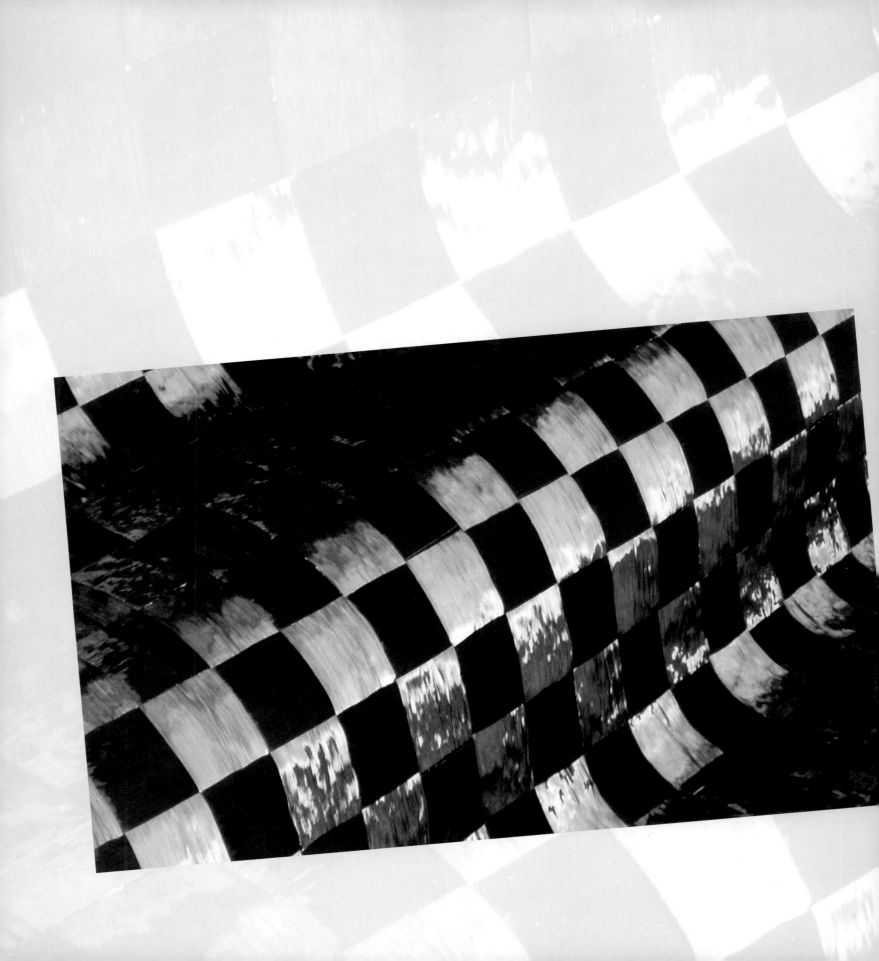

Materials

Why is material innovation such an important focus of creativity in the field of textiles today? One explanation is that a period of unprecedented innovation has occurred as a new area of research expertise – material science – has emerged through the collaboration and transfer of expertise between the hitherto discrete disciplines of electronics, computing, chemistry, engineering and biology. As a result, we are living through a period of unprecedented material innovation that looks set to change the role and purpose of fabric in our lives.

Many of the materials surveyed in this chapter remain at an experimental stage and have yet to be put into manufacture. They arouse a sense of being at the threshold of a new world full of possibility, one step over which (if only we could decide on the right direction) could put a new way of life within our grasp. In contrast to the aspirations of the laboratory-based research carried out by the scientific community, the growth of material awareness among the design community may be seen as a levelling influence. Their work is mainly concerned with the consequences of the manufacture and disposal of commonplace materials and fabrics – which are out there and having an impact in the real world. To date, much of their work has been focused on recycling: they are concerned not with the potential of new technological combinations, but with the technical problems of disaggregation and of returning fibres, chemicals and dyestuffs to the earth. It is a perspective that reminds us that the environmental impacts of nanotechnology – an area that is generating particular excitement – have yet to be seriously studied.

Oxeon TeXtreme (2002) manufactured by Oxeon, Sweden, is a reinforcement fabric woven from tapes made from either carbon fibre, aramid fibre, boron or liquid ceramics.

The design enables weight reductions and speeds up composite manufacture.

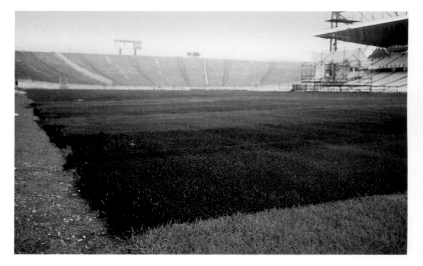

Nanotechnology and Surface Design

Nanotechnology is a field of material design where the smallest man-made devices encounter the atoms and molecules of the natural world (for comparative purposes, a nanometre is a billionth of a metre, the diameter of an atom is about a quarter of a nanometre, the average diameter of a human hair is 10,000 nanometres). It has the potential to bring about a revolution in surface design because it promises to take the imitation of natural materials to an advanced level of precision. Although working at the nanoscale has been with us for some time, this field was boosted by the development of atomic-scale probes in the 1980s (the scanning tunnelling microscope in 1981 and the atomic force microscope in 1986). Both use a needle or probe, which is mounted on a cantilever, as an electrode to provide an image of the configurations of atoms and molecules on the surface of materials. Imagine the needle on an old-fashioned record player: in crude terms, the way these probes trace the profile of materials is similar. The contrast with traditional techniques of chemical analysis, which reveal the chemical ingredients of materials by dissolving the sample, could not be greater.

These developments have the potential to inspire huge advances in the precision engineering of textile surfaces by improving our understanding of the character of biological material surfaces at the nanoscale. This is significant in two ways: firstly, because they reveal the nanoscale structural design elements that condition the overall behaviour of a given natural material and secondly, because this is the scale at which molecular biology takes place; in other words, it promises to help us to understand how these features are produced in the natural world. Billions of dollars are being invested in the United States, Japan and Europe with China keen to participate as well.

The second reason that people are excited about nanotechnology is because it is a scale (in terms of the ratio between surface area and volume) at which materials start to exhibit strikingly different physical and chemical properties. Graphite, for example, is usually brittle, but becomes pliable and conductive at the nanoscale, enabling self-assembled carbon fibres to be woven into yarn and potentially, cost permitting, into conductive fabrics. Silver, normally slow to tarnish, develops catalytic and anti-bacterial properties at the nanoscale which has already given it a vital role in the development of wound dressings and protective medical garments that can impede the spread of superbugs such as MRSA. Titanium dioxide particles can be catalysed by the sun to decompose stains, bad smells or viruses. Current applications of nanotechnology to fabric range from the trivial, such as bouncier tennis balls, to labour-saving fabrics that are wrinkle free, stain resistant and can shed dirt at lower temperatures, to nano meshes in water purification systems that can filter out harmful viruses such as polio or the bacteria that cause gastroenteritis: a huge potential for the developing world.

Secumat, Naue GmbH (Germany), has emerged as a world leader in the field of geotextiles. Secumat is a non-woven three-dimensional mat made of polymer monofilaments which encourages plant growth and prevents erosion on steep slopes. It has been successfully used on a football stadium in Paris.

Corpo Nove/Grado Zero Espace (Italy), 2003 (below). Liquid ceramics are normally used as an insulating material in the aerospace industries. However, clothing fabrics can also be treated in order to insulate the wearer from extreme weather conditions.

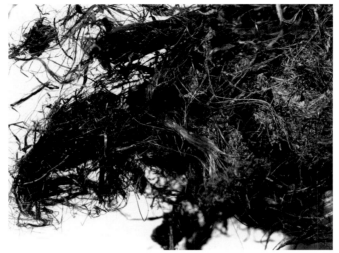

Corpo Nove/Grado Zero Espace R and D (Italy) have experimented with extracting fibres from nettles (left), peat (centre, right) and even tobacco leaves. Nettle is similar to hemp and flax, but is harder than hemp to extract, although scientists working at Grado Zero claim that they have devised a new method that may facilitate its manufacture.

Carbon nanotubes (bottom left) are one of the most promising new materials in textile science. As well as being conductors of heat and electricity, these sub-microscopic carbon fibres are light, strong and very flexible, although each one is only 10 to 50 nanometres in diameter. A research team led by Gordon Wallace from Australia's Commonwealth Scientific and Research Organization (CSIRO)'s Division of Textile and Fibre developed this conducting polymer fibre.

A three-dimensional woven beam made by Biteam (Sweden) from carbon fibres (below, right). Delamination is a fundamental problem with the use of fibres in composite materials. Biteam's use of three-dimensional weaving enables it to create lighter, stronger bespoke structural components for aircraft construction.

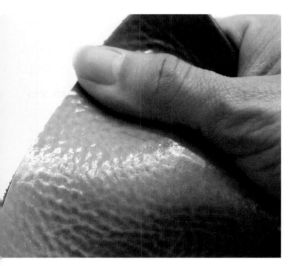

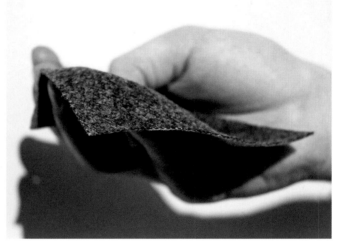

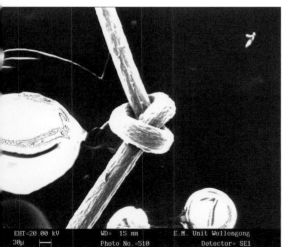

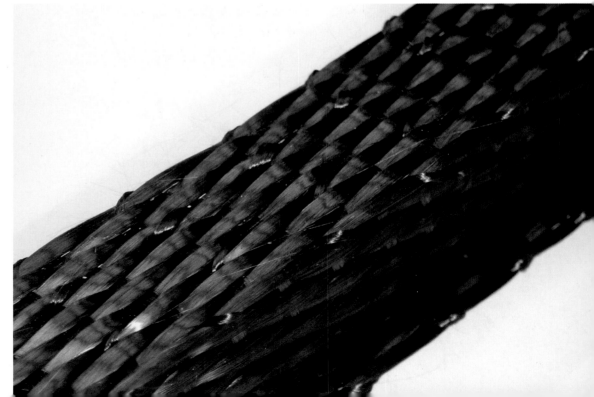

NANOTECHNOLOGY AND SURFACE DESIGN

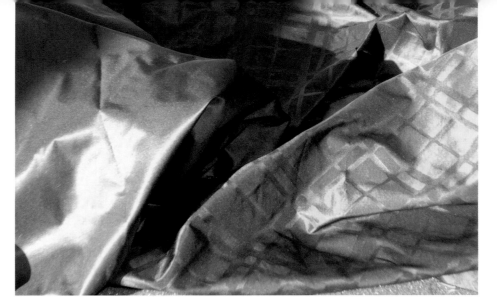

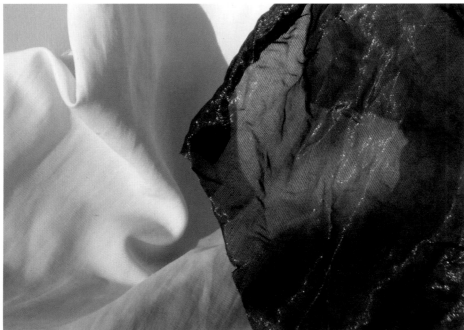

Schoeller Textil AG, Switzerland, make
fashion fabrics that are breathable and
water and wind repellant. *Copper* (above),
polyester, PU and polyamide. *Misty* (left),
10% metallic yarn, 30% elasthane and 60%
polyamide. *Jeans Steel* (below), 5% elasthane,
20% polyamide, 30% cotton and 45%
metallic yarn. A 2way stretch fabric.

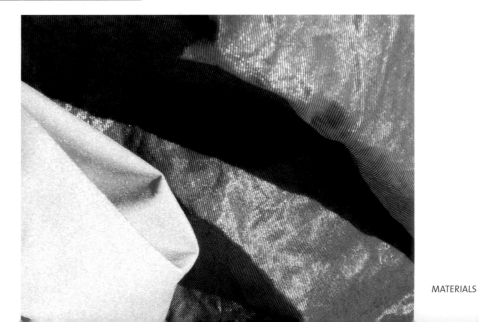

Sophie Roet, *Metal Dress*, 2001. CS-Interglas normally produce coated glass fibre fabrics for industrial and architectural applications. Roet adapted their techniques to produce fabrics suitable for fashion or interior applications. Silks, cotton and felt are layered with a metallic sheeting, neoprene glues and natural resin to produce fabrics that can be manipulated into three-dimensional forms by hand.

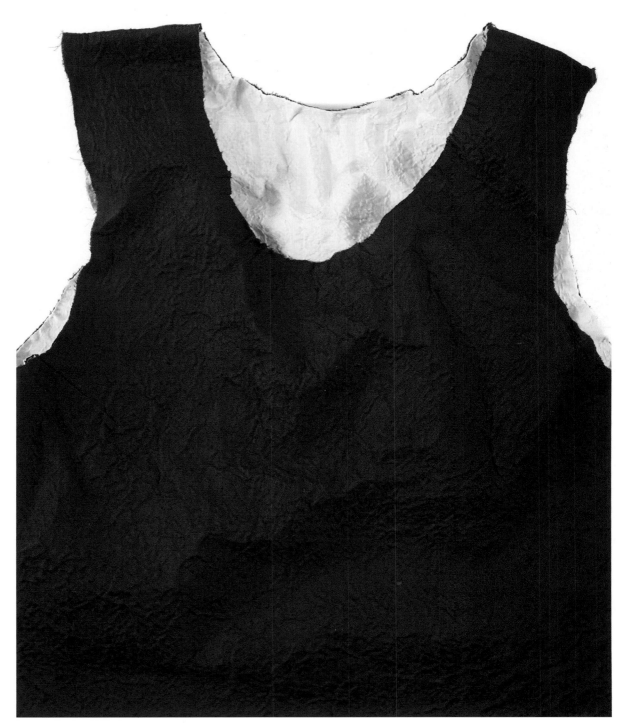

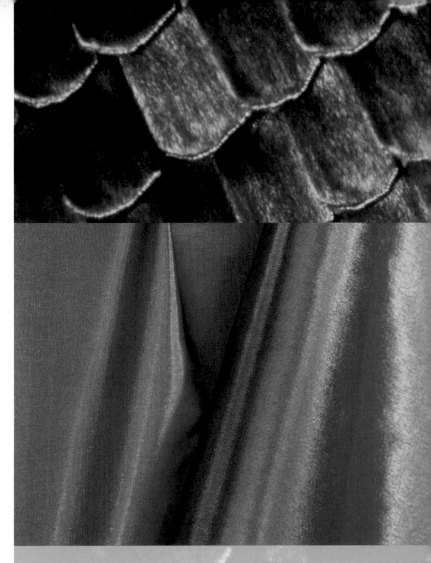

Coloured scanning electron micrograph of the male Morpho butterfly found in Brazil. The tiny overlapping scales that cover the butterfly's wing are transparent, but refract and reflect light to different extents to produce a shimmering blue-green appearance which is attractive to females.

Fibres with Tactile, Aural and Optical Properties

In the late 1980s, the search for synthetic fabrics with improved aesthetic and tactile qualities – which would overcome the shortcomings of the first generation of synthetics – led to the production of highly engineered polyester microfibres. It was found that by giving these fibres a *structure* the surface properties of the final textile could be improved. In Japan, the textile industry invested in a substantial amount of research and development funding in this. Initially they managed to create polyester fabrics that could imitate the scroop (the distinctive rasping rustle) of silk, or were better able to absorb and diffuse sweat by virtue of having perforations etched along the surface of the fibre. But in the 1990s a new generation of fabrics emerged, for example, Kuraray's 'angel-skin' fabric – a velvet made from polyester and cotton microfibres. Collectively they were called *Shin Gosen* or *Shin Shin Gosen* (second or third generation synthetic fibres), which came to convey the idea that their technologically enhanced aesthetic qualities transcended the mere mimesis of natural materials such as silk.

Yet by the late 1990s textile technologists were once again studying biological materials to draw out the potential of new yarn manufacturing technologies. In 2000 the Japanese company Teijin, in collaboration with the Japanese car manufacturer Nissan, launched a new product that mimicked the 'roof tile' arrangement of scales of cuticle, a near transparent polymeric protein (similar to fingernails), that gives the wings of Morpho butterflies their brilliant hue. With Morphotex they created a fibre that is *coloured by structure* as opposed to pigments or dyes. It is made up of multiple nanoscale layers of polyester and nylon: the multi-layer optical interference produces changes in colour, from blue to purple, red and green. Whereas scientists had hitherto tried to develop synthetic fibres with improved tactile, aural, or tensile qualities this was the first time that a fibre with specific optical properties had been designed: a hugely significant development.

In the 1990s Japan became famous for engineering synthetic fibres with enhanced tactile and acoustic properties. Attention then switched to optical characteristics and in 2003 Japanese textile giant Teijin opened a plant for the commercial production of its polychromic fibre, Morphotex. Morphotex is a fibre that is not coloured by pigment or dye, but instead by tiny synthetic layers along the surface of each fibre which cause light interference. Taking their inspiration from the brilliant iridescent blues and green of the male Morpho butterfly's wings, Morphotex mimics the roof tile arrangement of layers of cuticle on the butterfly's wings. The fibre was the product of a seven-year research programme in collaboration with Tanaka Kinzoku Kogyo.

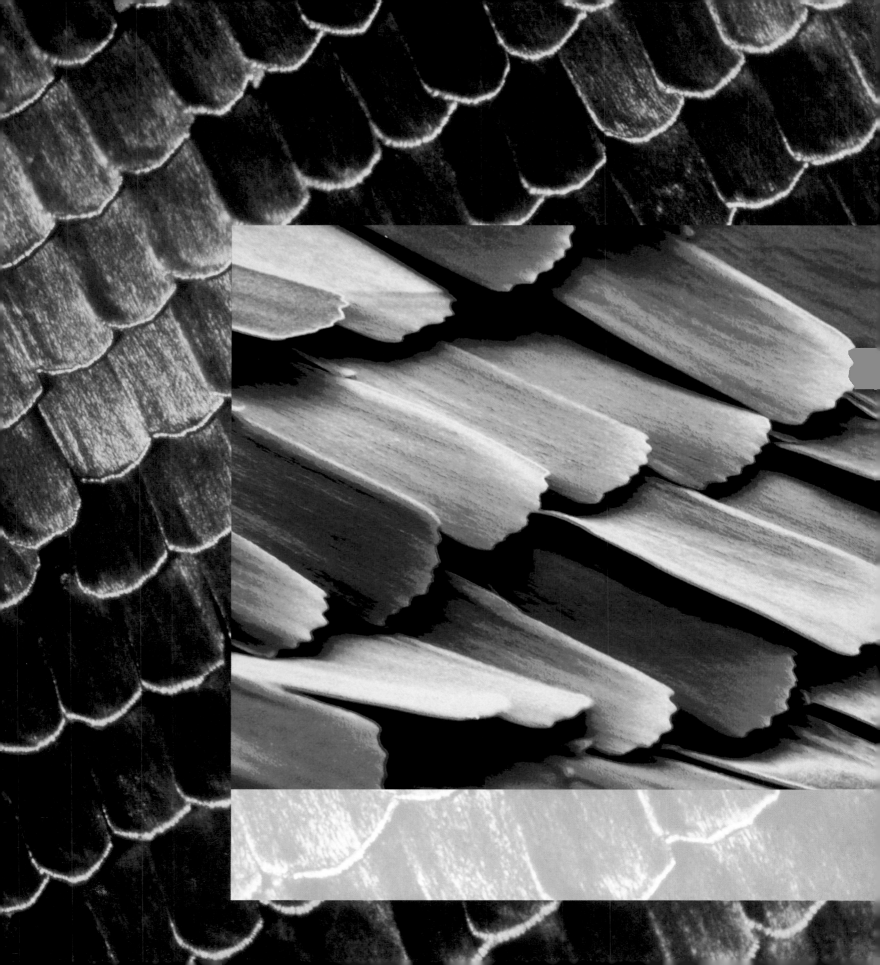

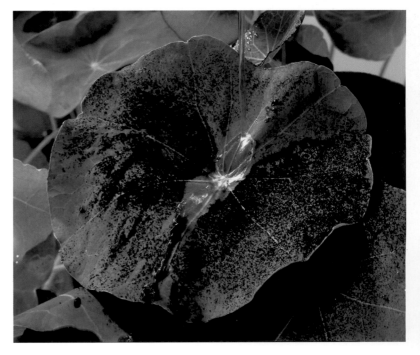

Biomimicry

Morphotex is a reminder that innovation in the field of textiles is not purely scientifically and technologically driven, but that innovation can also be inspired by nature. Biomimicry does not see nature as a resource of raw materials, but rather seeks to learn from the way natural materials are formed. Biomimicry studies these materials and takes inspiration from them to solve contemporary problems. One of its chief advocates, Janine Benyus, states: 'Nature has been innovating for 38 billion years, which has given it enough time to establish what works and what doesn't.'

The development of Velcro by the Swiss engineer George de Mestral was inspired by the hooks of burdock burrs. In 1975 the German botanist Wilhelm Barthlott discovered the self-cleaning properties of nasturtium and lotus leaves. Although the surfaces of both leaves feel smooth, studies with an electron microscope revealed that they have a rough micro-texture comprised of 'teeth' made from wax crystals. The combination of the wax and this roughness causes water to bead up and roll off the leaf's surface carrying dirt with it. Over twenty years later, in 1997, when advances in nanotechnology made it possible, Barthlott devised a technical analogue of this process, which he patented under the term lotus-effect. He has recently created a lotus-effect spray that can be applied to clothing and footwear with the German chemical company BASF. Textile manufacturers have developed similar technologies. The Swiss company Schoeller, who produce a range of high-tech fabrics for skiwear, have recently launched a self-cleaning fabric that uses nanospheres, while Burlington's Nano-tex uses nano-whiskers to produce a similar effect.

The development of the lotus-effect shows that the mimesis of nature is not static. It is a process that evolves in tandem with technological change: it was Japan's expertise in fibre technology that led to the development of Morphotex. Likewise, the development of new fabrics can encourage scientists towards new discoveries in the natural world which may, in turn, prompt the development of new material technologies. Since the 1990s, the interest in the synthetics industry's performance fibres, for example, has made biologists and research chemists look for high-performing materials in the natural world. And in the past decade as much effort has been poured into emulating the extraordinary properties of spider silk as was formerly devoted to mimicking silkworm silk.

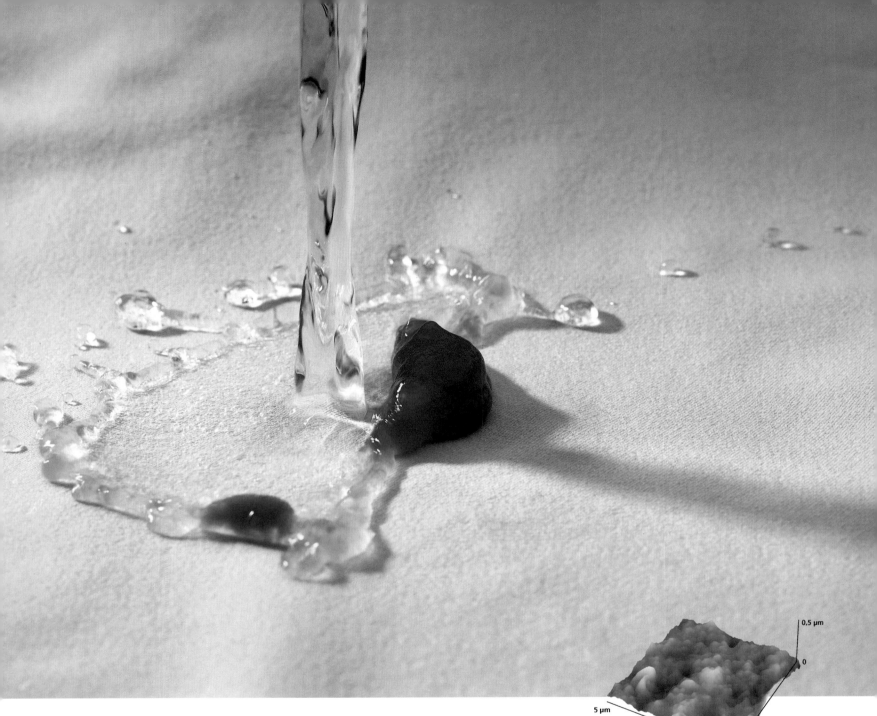

Plants and animals can inspire sophisticated engineering. In the 1970s the German botanist William Barthlott discovered that the self-cleaning properties of lotus and nasturtium leaves was not caused by their smoothness, but by the miniature spicules on their surfaces which caused water to bead up and roll off them. In 2001 Schoeller Textil AG, Switzerland, launched NanoSphere, a fabric coating capable of repelling water, oil and even honey, but it does not affect the way the fabric feels or moves. As atomic resonance imaging shows, the coating matrix fixes nanoscale particles of silica in such a way as to ensure that they are firmly anchored into the surface of the fabric.

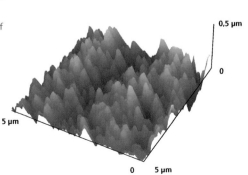

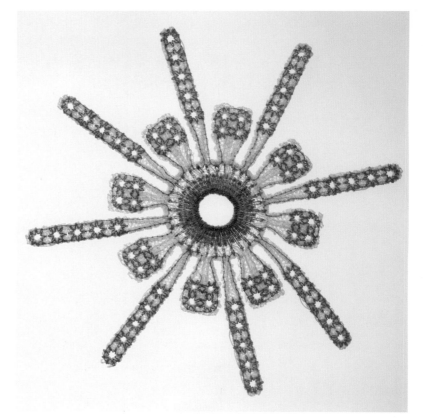

Medical Textiles

Spiders are believed to have spun silk for some 400 million years, yet their silk may well become the natural fibre of the future. Even if highly engineered synthetic fibres can surpass it in terms of certain *individual* properties, spider silk has the potential to outstrip existing oil-based polymers because it *combines* many different useful characteristics. The silk is light, stretchy and strong: it is tougher than Kevlar and not only five times stronger than tensile steel, but also six times lighter; it is as elastic as nylon and it can also be made magnetic and conductive; and it is stable at high temperatures. Its potential applications range from lightweight, bulletproof vests to suspension bridges and to nerve, tendon and bone repair. The problem is how to access sufficient quantities: since spiders are cannibalistic, spider farms are out of the question.

Scientists have attempted to produce both synthetic and genetically engineered analogues of spider silk. In Canada *spidroin* (spider silk protein) has been extracted from the udders of genetically modified goats, but this substance has lacked the mechanical properties of the natural material. More recent research by Professor Paula Hammond, a research director of the Institute for Soldier Nanotechnologies at MIT, has suggested that the unique physical properties of spider silk may be explained by studying its chemical structure. It is comprised of two active components: small crystalline rafts that are suspended in a more elastic matrix (which may itself be comprised of a sandwich of partially aligned polymers), a combination that serves to give this material its resilience. Her team is attempting to develop synthetic analogues of spider silk that may be cheaply made into military uniforms.

Yet it is the highly energy efficient way in which spiders produce silk at room temperature that makes them extraordinary. According to two Oxford zoologists, Dr David Knight and Professor Fritz Vollrath, high-performance spider silk fibres may eventually replace oil-based polymers such as aramids like DuPont's Kevlar or the new high-performance aramid being developed with Magellan Systems M5, which derive their tensile and compressive strength and, in the case of Magellan its fire-resistant properties, from being manufactured at high temperatures in vats of acid and require treatment with toxic organic solvents.

Embroidered surgical implants by Ellis Developments (UK). Based in Nottingham, Ellis Developments specializes in the design and development of textiles for engineering and medical applications. Bespoke textile grafts, machine embroidered on soluble cloth were used in the world's first operation to insert an artificial clavicle in 2003.

They argue that the physical properties of spider silk may be better understood by studying the way spider silk proteins fold and crystallize as they are secreted and spun from within the spider's spinneret in an aqueous solution. As Vollrath observes: 'because the "spinning dope" (the material from which silk is spun) is liquid crystalline, spiders can draw it during extrusion into a hardened fibre using minimal forces. This involves an unusual process whereby the silk initially solidifies and forms *within* the spider's spinning duct prior to being extruded from its spinneret and coming into contact with the air.' They have recently set up a company to develop a mechanical spinning process that will convert other silk proteins found in silkworm silk, and even rice, by mimicking the way in which spiders secrete and spin. The process is expensive and currently materials are only produced for biomedical applications.

Whether or not their invention becomes as important to the development of spinning technology in the 21st century as Richard Arkwright's Spinning Jenny in the 18th, the debate is fascinating because it is an example of the growing hope that biomimesis (understood here in the broadest terms possible, that is, as the mimesis of not merely biological forms but of biological processes and systems) may yet transform foundering textile industries in the West.

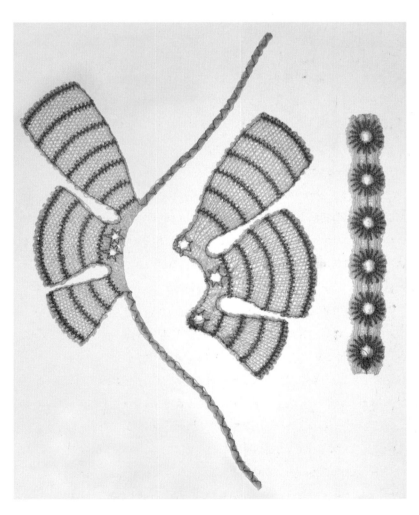

Surgeons use machine-embroidered textile grafts as a form of scaffolding to promote nerve and muscle repair. The inter-vertebral implants pictured here look beautiful, but their design serves a strictly functional purpose. One advantage of embroidery is that threads can be arranged in multiple directions and owing to the flexibility of CAD/CAM can easily be tailored to fit the patient. The rotary cuff pictured here was custom designed for a patient who had a tumour removed from his shoulder: the design was subsequently adapted to help muscles attach themselves to his humerus.

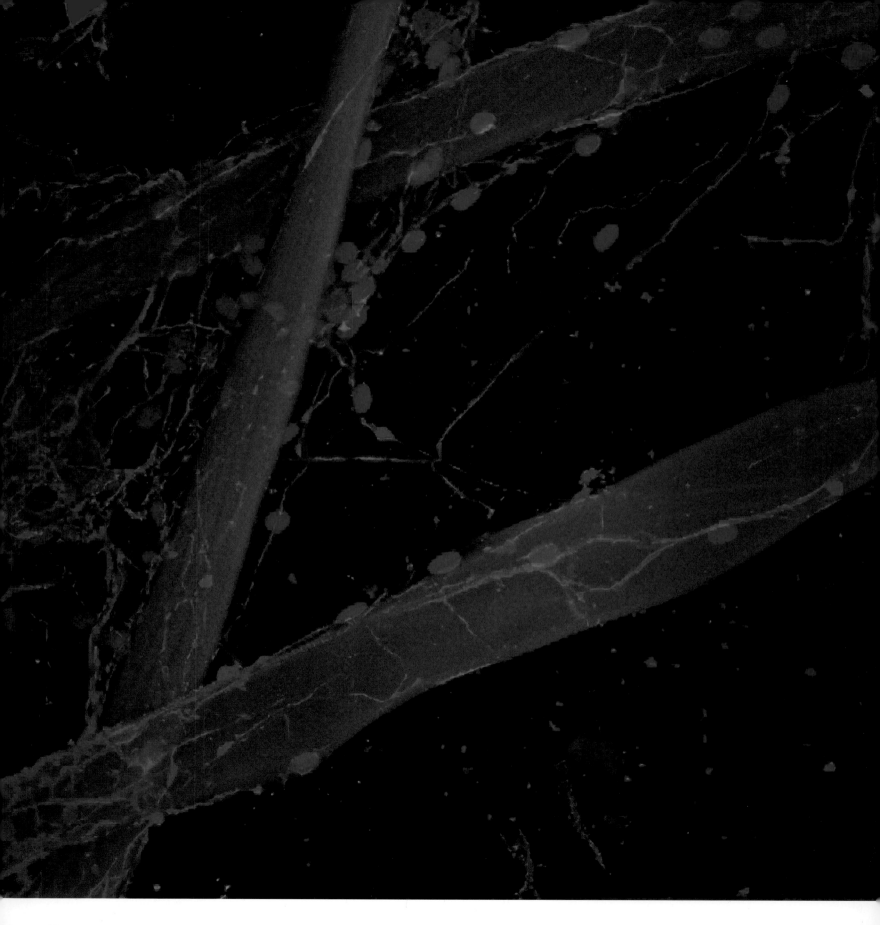

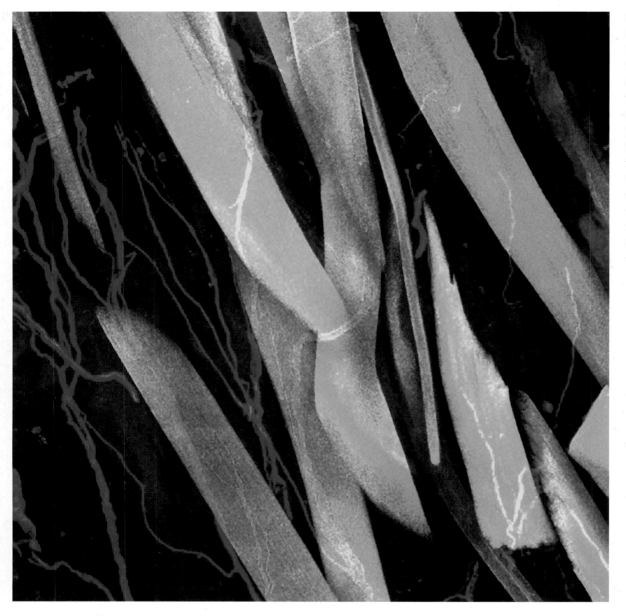

Spidrex was developed by Oxford Biomaterials, manned by staff from the Department of Zoology at Oxford University, in 2003. Oxford Biomaterials have developed a means of giving silkworm silk some of the amazing mechanical properties of spider dragline silk by employing a spinning process that mimics the precise manner in which spiders secrete and draw down their silk. Although it can only be manufactured in small quantities at the moment, Spidrex has many potential medical applications, including nerve regeneration for spinal injuries. The images show axons of the spinal chord (in red) regenerating on lengths of Spidrex.

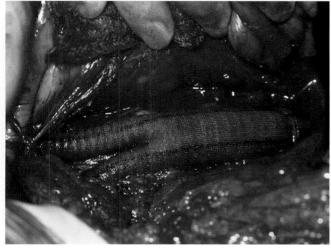

Example of a Dacron implant being used to fix an aortic aneurysm.

Clothing and Protection

Since 2001 American technology has been shaped by the so-called War on Terror. Homeland security now tops the list of funding prerogatives for the US Research and Development budget. Characteristically, Americans are turning to new technologies to provide a solution to problems of security. Yet even before 9/11 the US Army and Navy had already embarked on an extensive research programme to augment the capacities of infantrymen through the use of computer wearables and e-textiles. Despite the development of unmanned military vehicles, the experience of recent conflict in the Gulf, Somalia, Afghanistan and Iraq has shown that ground troops are still required to occupy a position in person. Accordingly, the US military began to fund scientific research that might enable them to fit out the infantry with 'smart uniforms' that could protect soldiers from ballistic and chemical attack, or from extreme weather conditions and perform basic triage when they were deployed as foot soldiers away from armoured vehicles or their support bases.

The Future Force Warrior Programme run by the US Army Natick Soldier Center envisages a future where a soldier's physical capacity will be enhanced by artificially powered exoskeletons (developed by the Bleek programme at the University of Berkeley, California) and actuators (textile muscles), where smart textiles embedded with sensors will protect the soldier from biochemical, nuclear and ferromagnetic armour ballistic attack and where computer wearables and e-textiles will enhance a soldier's vision and provide on-field information sourced from satellites and unmanned aircraft. It has attracted a huge amount of publicity partly, one suspects, because it engages with popular science fiction characters such as the Bionic Man, the Terminator, cyborgs and robots. The similarities are not coincidental. In fact, the Future Force Warrior is both a conceptual and public relations exercise that aims to raise public support for defence spending as well as stirring up the imagination and provoking public debate and dialogue on how these technologies and concepts might be able to help soldiers in the future. It is a strategy that enables the US Army to draw upon the work of leading scientists in the public domain whose work by definition needs to be open to public scrutiny. In terms of the development of textile research in the United States, this programme is of immense importance since it attracts generous funding, which currently exceeds comparable civilian initiatives.

One of the most enduringly influential prototypes for a smart uniform was developed by Indian-born Sundaresan Jayaraman, Professor of Textile and Fibre Engineering at the Georgia Technology Institute. He responded to an appeal put out by the US Navy in 1996;

'The Georgia Tech Wearable Motherboard' developed by Sundaresan Jayaraman, 1996–1998, at the Georgia Technology Institute (USA) was internationally heralded as a major step towards integrating sensing technology within clothing. This seamless garment is woven from a stretchy, body-hugging fabric (spandex and polypropylene), which incorporates conductive fibres (polyethylene with a copper core and from nylon doped in inorganic particles), a static dissipating element and a long plastic fibre optic filament that curls around the body of the wearer. They are connected to a personal status monitor. Jayaraman is pictured wearing his prototype – it is illuminated and ready to detect penetration by a bullet. The sensors can alert firemen to noxious fumes or help parents monitor a baby's heartbeat.

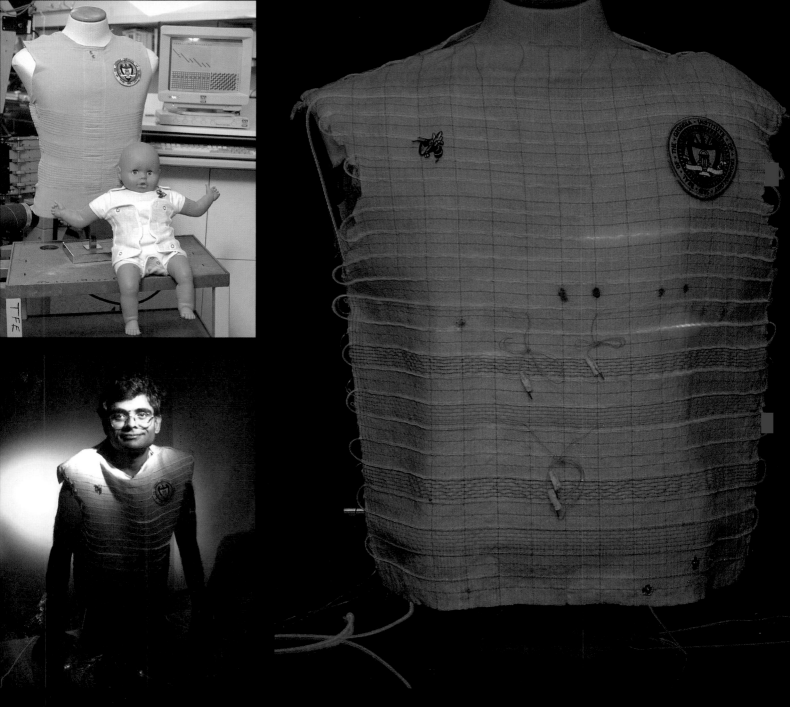

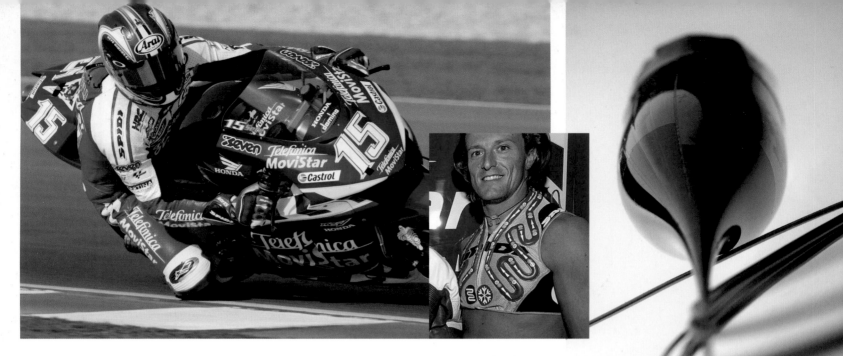

'The Georgia Tech Wearable Motherboard' was the first garment to incorporate both fibre optics and conductive fibres into a garment that could be used to monitor the health of soldiers on the battlefield. Because it is woven from a single piece of fabric, a signal could pass along an optical fibre that formed a continuous loop around the body of the wearer and was connected to a monitor worn at the hip. The shirt could be used to monitor ballistic attack. If the optical fibre was damaged (by a bullet, for example) the monitor would detect the interruption of the signal and could convey this information back to base. Further sensors attached to the body of the soldier and to conductive threads could be used to monitor oxygen levels.

Jayaraman's prototype has led to significant developments in the field and it has inspired the manufacture of a number of similar devices for civilian use in Europe, Japan and South Korea. These range from health-monitoring vests for babies at risk of cot death, or perhaps more worryingly, a sensing shirt for the elderly whose health can be monitored 'via a secure internet connection'. Yet by far the most significant development has occurred at MIT. In 2002, the US military embarked on a defensive campaign based on the development of new materials for

textiles. They donated $50 million to set up a five-year research programme – the Institute for Soldier Nanotechnologies. Its aim was to create a futuristic battle suit. Ferromagnetic materials could be used to engineer a form of liquid armour that would be as thin and flexible as a T-shirt in one state, but which could transform into hardened armour as needed once a magnetic impulse was applied. Hollow fibres about 100 microns wide filled with microcapsules contain ferromagnetic particles that could be activated to stiffen when exposed to a magnetic impulse. A third innovation being developed is actuators (muscle-like fabric), fibres comprised of ribbons of polymer hinges that can bend, tighten and relax in response to electrical impulses, that could potentially boost a soldier's muscle lifting capacity by 25 to 30 per cent.

However, the main reason that MIT attracted government funding to establish its institute was the level of sophistication that had been reached in the development of conductive fabrics with enhanced optical properties. Clothing people in optical fibres and traditional wiring had presented a number of technical challenges. If high-power optical fibres are bent then their cores, which are typically made of glass or silica, will break. Likewise, metal wiring that does not bend

In 2006 the McLaren team sported self-cooling suits to help mechanics and motorcyclists perform in extreme weather conditions. The suit features a miniaturized air-conditioning system developed by Grado Zero Espace, Italy, in conjunction with the European Space Agency Technology Transfer Programme.

In 2004 Yoel Fink and his colleagues at MIT (USA) developed a fibre drawing technique to create materials with enhanced optical properties. Pictured here is the preform composed of conductive, semi-conductive and insulating materials which is heated in a furnace and then drawn into a fibre.

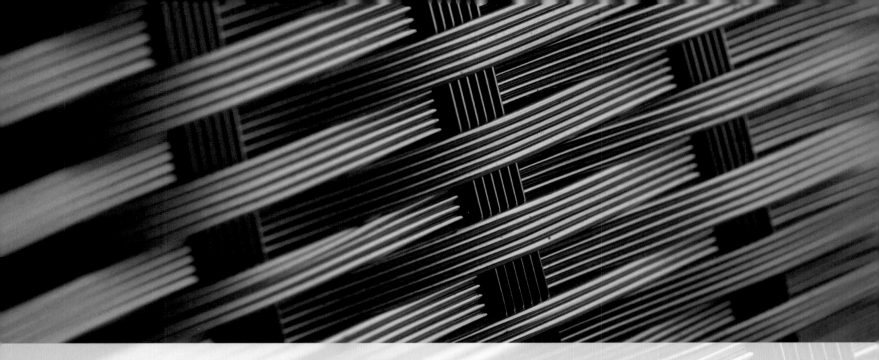

back becomes fatigued. In 2002, researchers at MIT, led by Israeli scientist Yoel Fink, created high-performance mirrors in the shape of hair-like flexible fibres that could be woven into cloth and cut to make clothes. Like Gutenberg's realization that a device similar to a wine press might serve to imprint moveable type, Fink's innovation involved combining the design of mirrors, semi-conductors and the innovative optical properties of Morphotex.

In 1998, roughly at the same time that Teijin were developing Morphotex, Fink created a 'perfect' mirror by microstructuring the *internal* surface of a fibre in a new way. Made of alternating layers of polystyrene and the rare metal element, tellurium, his 'perfect mirror' combined the advantages of a conventional metallic mirror with those of a dielectric mirror. The latter is a mirror that is comprised of alternating layers of non-metallic material that can be tuned to reflect certain wavelengths of light, thereby allowing much greater control over the mirrors reflectivity, but can only reflect light from a limited number of angles. Fink's perfect mirror not only reflects light from all angles, but can also be tuned to reflect certain wavelengths while transmitting others.

Helped by the young Turkish physicist Mehmet Bayindir, among others, Fink has developed two significantly novel fibres out of this research. They are a classic example of dual-purpose technology, whereby technologies made to serve military requirements are developed to meet civilian needs as well. In instances where Fink's nanostructured sheath lines the inner core of the fibre with the semiconductors wrapped around it promises significant advances in laser surgery and telecommunications. And, on the other hand, if the nanostructured sheath is placed on the fibre's *surface*, so that it can achieve some contact with the semi-conductive material at its core, it can be used to create an interactive fabric interface: a sophisticated optical device. This promises to pave the way for a new fabric computer interface that can be activated by infra-red light.

Such fibres could also be incorporated in the fabric of a battlesuit, or a sheet of paper where they could reflect an infra-red bar code to identify a soldier, or be made to change the colour they reflect for camouflage purposes, or be tuned to reflect radiation in the event of a nuclear attack. The design of fibres with optical properties has been taken to an entirely new level.

Spectrometric Fabric developed by Yoel Fink, MIT (USA). In 2004 Fink and his research team from the Photonic Bandgap Fibers and Devices Group achieved a breakthrough in optical design, materials development and fibre manufacturing techniques. This prototype fabric can not only sense light, but can also potentially analyse its colours. The fabric is composed of light-sensitive composite fibres. Each fibre has separate channels for transmitting light and electrical currents. In 1998 Fink developed high-performance mirrors in the shape of hair-like synthetic fibres. The spectrometric fabric draws upon this research. Potential applications include light-sensitive flexible fabric computer screens or protective military clothing.

An ongoing ambition of military
technologists is to create technologically
enhanced camouflage that would cloak
soldiers with invisibility. As part of the
Future Warrior Program researchers at
the US Army Soldier Systems Centre
at Natick have tried to develop uniforms
made from fibre optics that would transmit
the appropriate camouflage imagery,
whereby a soldier standing in front of a
brick wall, for example, would be able to
get his uniform to project a similar surface
photographic visualization.

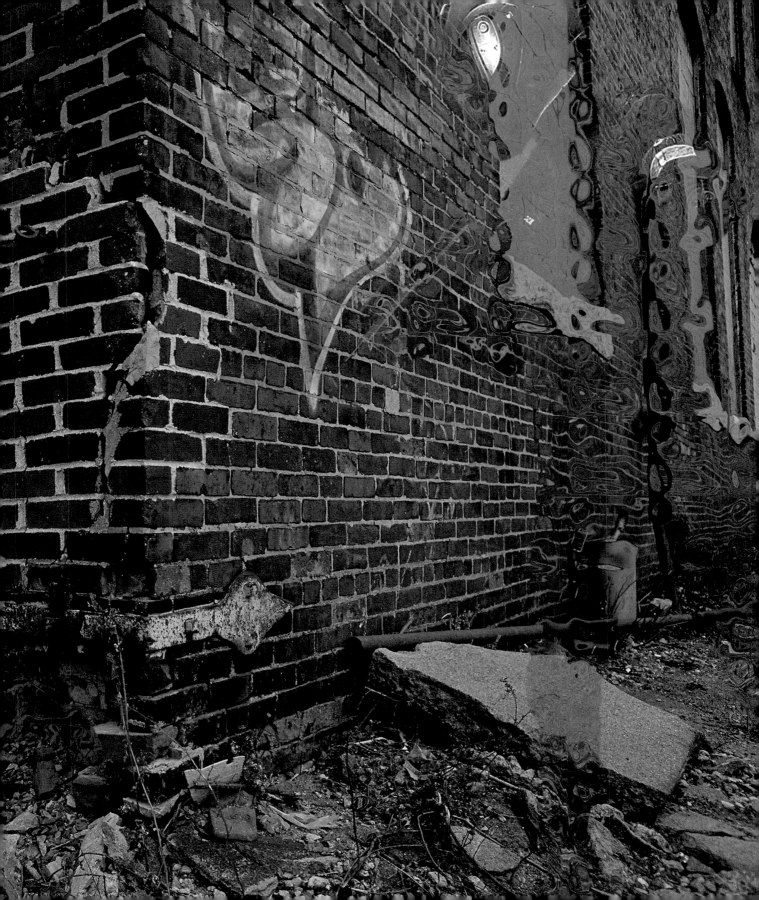

Clothing by Elisabeth de Senneville (France) with Flexible LED Screens (10 x 7 cm in size) that have been connected to a battery with a four-hour charge life. In 2004 a research team led by Emeric Mourot at France Telecom developed working prototypes of flexible colour screens that were connected to the internet via blue tooth technology. To make the display LEDs were soldered onto a flexible circuit board which was then packaged into a fabric sandwich.

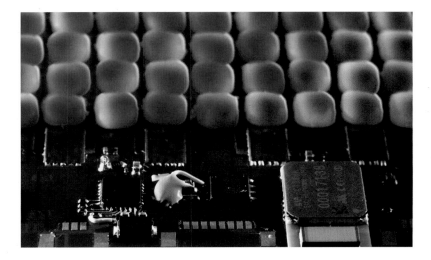

Fabric Robots and the Fabric Computer

The development of textile-based digital displays may be affected significantly by Fink's innovative fibre technologies. Emeric Mourot, Director of the research and development team at France Telecom, has led two different approaches that address difficulties with clothing-based displays. In 2001 flexible displays (display screens) were successfully integrated into fabrics by incorporating fibre optics into cloth. They created a screen matrix by weaving fibre optics and classic yarns into a specific structure. The optical fibres were able to illuminate specific target units of this matrix by virtue of small perforations along the surface of the fibre optic cable. As a result of this design Mourot's team won the innovation award at Techtextil/Avantex 2002 (the Frankfurt-based trade fair for e-textiles), although it did not prove washing-machine friendly so in 2004 they developed a much smaller flexible LED screen that could be integrated into the pocket of an item of clothing and could be linked via bluetooth technology to mobile phones or the internet.

There is also already considerable commercial involvement in sensors, another area of e-textiles. The British company Eleksen have developed a touch sensor made from a five-layer fabric sandwich. Two layers of carbon-fibre conductive fabric encase a three-layer sandwich of semi-conductive fabric interleaved by an insulating mesh, forming a flexible touch sensor that conducts electricity when it is stroked or compressed. The accuracy of Eleksen sensors is derived from measuring the change in voltage between the top and bottom layers. Applications have ranged from the development of a flexible computer keyboard, which can be attached to a palm-held computer and then rolled up in a pocket, to a series of touch-sensitive key pads for an MP3 portable music player which has been incorporated within a ski jacket.

New Zealand engineer Brian Russell has launched a small start-up company, Zephyr Technology, to produce a textile pressure sensor called iMAT. In this case a matrix of linked carbon cells is ink-jet printed onto sheets of mylar which are sandwiched together. The two sheets generate electrical field effects when they move or stretch relative to each other. Additional electronics and software can, in turn, interpret these effects in terms of pressure and movement. A number of applications are possible – one currently being explored incorporates the material into cushions designed for wheelchair users and the occupants of hospital beds, where the points of extended physical pressure that lead to the development of sores can be monitored.

All these innovations can be defined as 'smart fabrics'. Fabrics of increasing sensitivity have emerged as the field of responsive polymer composites has expanded with the development of nanotechnology.

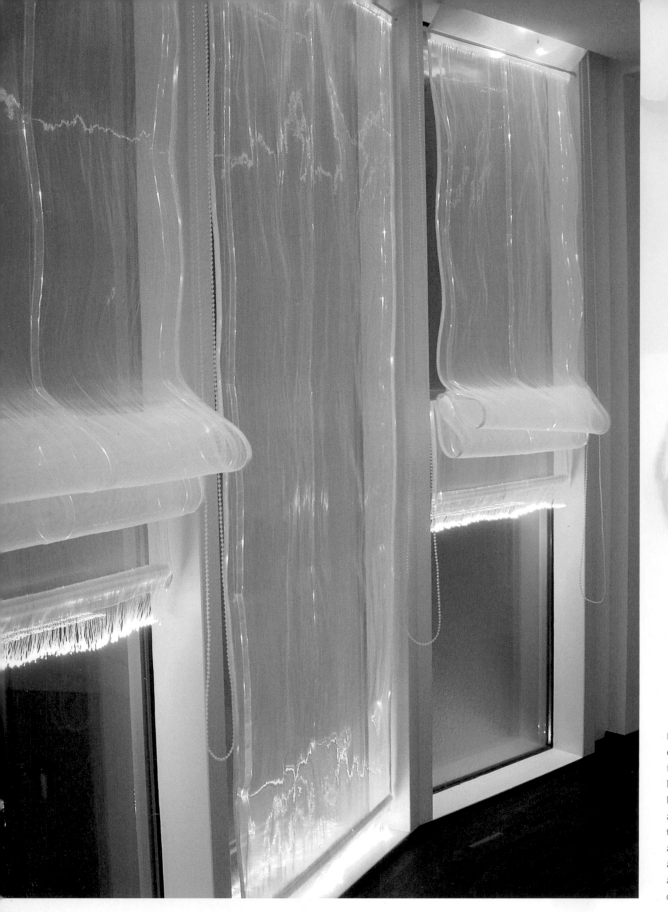

Lichtextil Luminex spa (Switzerland). Light-emitting diodes and fibre optics have been in commercial production since the 1970s, however, it is only recently that they have been used to illumine optical fibres which are woven into cloth. Curtains are attached to a transformer plugged into the wall and clothes made from these fabrics are attached to a battery. The cloth can be cut and washed in a washing machine on the delicates cycle.

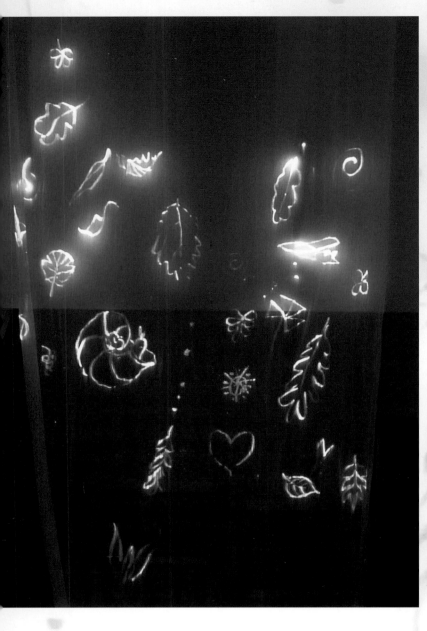

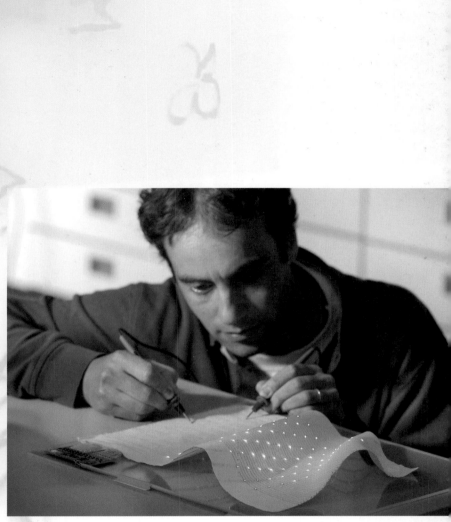

An early prototype of a photonic textile by Philips (Netherlands), 2005, which shows how engineers have succeeded in integrating flexible arrays of multicolored LEDs into fabrics. Their lumalive textile garments were on show in 2006.

The British company Eleksen's core technology is the touch-sensitive textile, ElekTex. ElekTex is a laminate of five fabric layers which are arranged to form a resistive touchpad. The sensor is contact activated: when touched, the layers are compressed together to form an electronic circuit. Eleksen launched a fabric keyboard in 2006 which has been followed by a small flexible screen.

Softswitch keypad developed by Softswitch Ltd (UK) for Burton apparel in 2005.

Zephyr Technology (New Zealand) are experts in the manufacture of pressure sensors. Here, a matrix of linked carbon cells has been printed on mylar. Two sheets in a sandwich generate electric field effects when they move or stretch relative to each other. Additional electronics and software can, in turn, interpret these effects in terms of pressure and movement. A number of applications are possible: one currently being explored incorporates this material into cushions designed for wheelchair users which can monitor their seating posture. The sensors could prevent bed sores by alerting the need for the user to shift position.

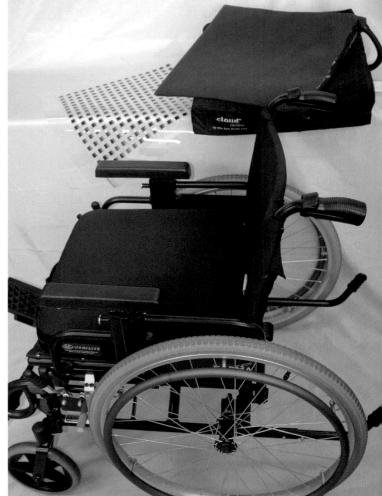

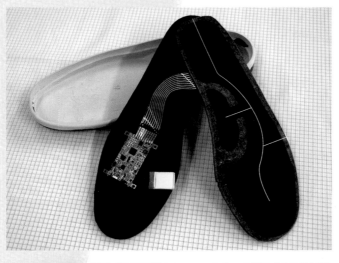

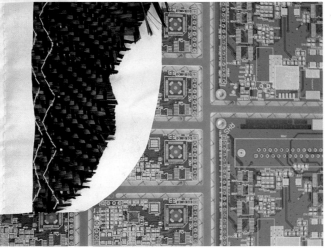

IMAT is a new pressure-sensing technology that uses electric-field measuring techniques to determine the distance between two surfaces. They are cheap to manufacture and can be used in a range of applications. Pictured here are two still lifes showing the important components of a pressure-sensing system: carbon mylar shoe inserts and a polyurethane foam compressible cushion radio that links hardware and circuit boards prior to manufacture.

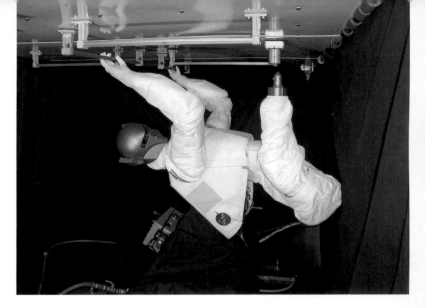

David Lussey, formerly an engineer working for the British Royal Air Force, developed a metallic particle with particular conductive properties. When these metallic particles are loaded in an elastomer, which is in turn sandwiched between layers of conductive and insulating material, they create an electrical insulator that can be turned into a metal-like conductor when a small force is applied. If coated onto a textile, it converts the textile into an electric switch that can be operated by finger pressure.

It is the shape of Lussey's particles that make the electrical properties of his composite material so unusual. The spikes of these particles are almost unimaginably small, similar in size to the tip on an atomic force microscope (approximately ten nanometres), and they enable the material to conduct electricity using the phenomenon of quantum tunnelling, whereby electrons pass through an energy barrier to cover short distances. It is as if someone hitting a tennis ball against a wall should occasionally find the ball passing through the wall's surface to reappear on the other side. It is an example of the way in which quantum mechanics, until recently the preserve of theoretical physics, has begun to be harnessed to speed up reactions between particles at very short distances. Lussey's Quantum Tunnelling Composite makes fabric so sensitive to its surroundings that it might almost be said to

have a number of human-like qualities: it can respond to touch, sound and heat, and it can 'smell' chemical vapours. NASA are using the Quantum Tunnelling Composite on the fingers of their robots to give them touch capability, and have also produced a sensitized textile glove to fit onto a robot hand.

Fabric sensors fall into the category of passive smart materials. Active smart materials, however, cannot only sense, but can also *respond* to their immediate environment. The Ukrainian scientist Sergiy Minko, who is Professor of Chemistry at Clarkson University in Potsdam New York, has developed a responsive polymer membrane that can encase polymer fibres to create a dynamic fabric that can alter its character in response to external stimulae. Responsive textiles using this technology can switch from ultrahydrophobic, or water repelling, to hydrophilic, water-absorbing. Responsive nano-membranes are tailored to open and close in response to external signals (such as acidity, salinity, biomolecules, or other chemicals that are used as stimuli). Such materials have many potential applications in developing protective clothing or in the development of membranes for water purification.

Shape memory materials, which take one form at a certain temperature and transform into another shape when heated, are not

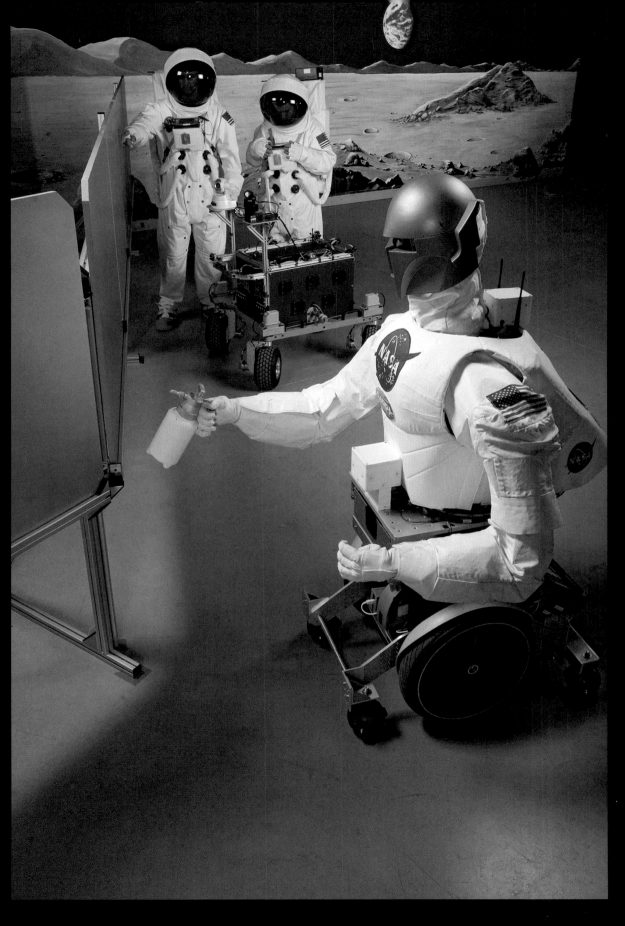

Robonaut B is the newer of two NASA robots used in recent hand-in-hand testing at the Johnson Space Center (JSC), Houston, with human beings to evaluate their shared ability to perform certain types of extravehicular activity.

Robonaut – which uses a head, torso, arms and dexterous hands to perform tasks using the same tools used by human spacewalkers – was fitted with a sensitized glove. NASA used QTC (a nano-tech Quantum Tunnelling electrically conductive polymer) developed by David Lussey of Peratech on the fingers of the glove to give them touch capability.

QTC has a number of human-like qualities: it can respond to touch, sound and heat and it can 'smell' vapours. It is an electrical insulator that can be turned into a metal-like conductor under very small forces. If it is coated onto a textile, it makes the textile into an electric switch that can be operated by finger pressure.

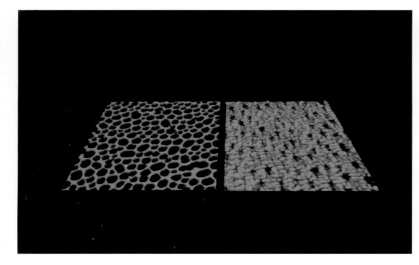

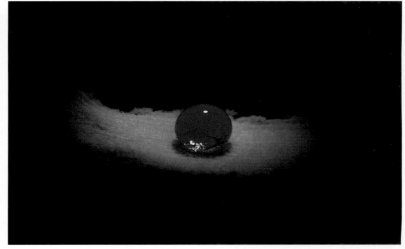

new: in fact shape memory alloys date back to the 1930s, but until now no shape memory plastics have been used in medical devices or proved to be biodegradable. In 2001 Andreas Lendlein of the Institute of Polymer Research in Aachen, Germany, together with MIT bio-engineer Robert Langer, developed a 'smart' plastic composed of two components: a hard segment and a 'switching' segment, which is activated at certain temperatures. The higher-temperature shape is the plastic's 'permanent' form, which it assumes after heating. They developed a company called mNemoscience to make coronary stents (the mesh tubes used to prop open blocked arteries) and tissue scaffolds for organ repair that could be tightly rolled up and introduced into the body using keyhole surgery. In 2005 the two scientists developed photosensitive, shape-changing biodegradable plastics, which are stable at high temperatures (50 degrees C), but can revert to a specific form when light of the correct wavelength is applied. This innovation might lead to a labour-saving fabric coating that could iron out creases in a shirt in response to heat or light and to car panels whose dents could be removed over night.

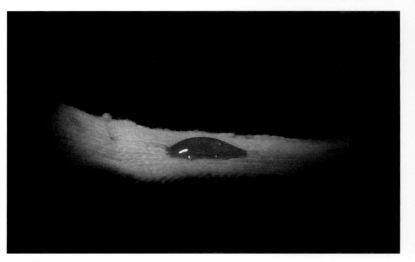

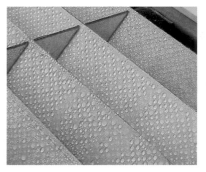

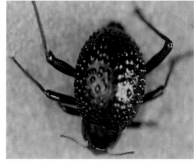

Sergiy Minko, Clarkson University, New York, 2006. A coloured drop of water shown initially a) on the surface of a smart textile and b) permeating the same piece of fabric demonstrates the remarkable properties of Minko's fabric which is capable of switching from an ultrahydrophobic (water repelling) to a hydrophilic (water permeable) state. Minko's fabric is an active smart material. Not only does this textile membrane allow sweat to evaporate from the body while protecting the wearer from rain, but its properties can also be switched so that it can be washed. The switching mechanism of the membrane can be rendered responsive to specific environmental triggers such as chemical toxins. The atomic force microscope images (above, left) show nanoscale membrane pores open in the air and closed when the fabric is submerged in water.

Chris Lawrence, QinetiQ (UK), *Printed Water Conducting Material*, 2001. Some species of desert beetle survive by drinking droplets of water extracted from desert fog. The surface of the Stenocara beetle's wings is covered with a pattern of hydrophilic bumps and waxy hydrophobic valleys. By angling their bodies towards the wind the beetles use their wings to attract minute droplets of water from the fog, which then bead up into larger droplets that flow down the waxy channels into the insect's mouth. In 2001, Chris Lawrence teamed up with Oxford zoologist Andrew Parker to develop biomimetic materials that would replicate these properties. They found that polyethylene printed with a precise arrangement of hydrophilic dots was far more efficient at harvesting water from fog.

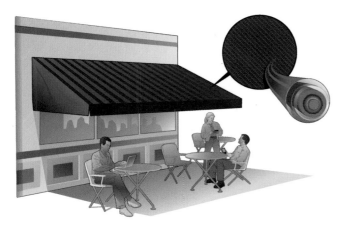

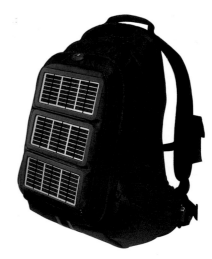

Ecological Fabrics

How to power protective clothing in the battlefield has long been an issue. Relying upon a battery pack poses difficulties, especially when the soldiers are sent away from their bases on long missions. According to an assessment made by DARPA (the United States Defense Advanced Research Projects Agency) in 2000, a soldier carrying a four-day power supply would have to leave behind 400 rounds of ammunitions and either four days' food rations or a protective mask and first aid kit. In the same year, the US military sponsored scientists at the Army Natick Soldier Center to develop advanced photovoltaic technology (solar cells are used to convert energy from the sun into electricity) for soldiers. Within months they had come up with a new way of making photovoltaic cells (PVCs) from nanoscale particles of titanium dioxide. Whereas existing silicon photovoltaics could only be applied to fragile materials such as glass, Konarka's photoreactive materials could be printed onto a range of flexible materials ranging from plastics to threads using ink-jet printing techniques developed for newspaper printing. At the moment photovoltaic cloth can only gather 4 per cent of the solar energy it receives from the sun, compared to silicon solar cells that can gather 18 per cent, however, it can harvest energy effectively from low-light frequencies; the manufacturing process is cheap and opens up the possibility.

Plastic photovoltaics are a successful example of the NASA effect, whereby significant technological innovations initially developed for the particular requirements of the US (and other) space programmes and the US military are adjusted to meet civilian needs. Yet it is an approach to innovation that can have its drawbacks. For example, although military funding has meant that a good deal of fundamental research into computer wearables has taken place, generating volumes of publicity over the past decade, no textiles incorporating electronic devices have been successfully commercialized in any great volume. In Europe a few electronic devices have been incorporated into specialist niche markets such as skiwear, equipment for outdoor rescue and medical textiles, but people have experienced difficulty in using laboratory ideas to develop new products. Textile designers and producers have built up the skills and awareness of people's differing needs over the years that electronic and microchip companies involved in this kind of research lack.

Sophisticated government strategies such as the Future Force Warrior Programme are both a symptom of, as well as a stimulant to, the growing public interest in material innovations. Consumer awareness of materials, or the provenance of textiles, is also beginning to echo what has already happened in the food industry, where people have

Detail showing the composition of a photovoltaic fibre. Light passes first through a transparent substrate, then through a transparent electrode and interacts with the active, composite polymeric core which contains both the photosensitive and semi-conducting materials that convert sunlight into electricity. Since 2005, Konarka Technologies (USA) has been working on the development of a photovoltaic cloth in conjunction with the Ecole Polytechnique Fédérale de Lausanne in Switzerland.

The energy-harvesting backpack developed by Voltaic Systems (USA), founded by Shayne McQuade in 2003, was greeted as a major step towards a radically distributed energy generation. This backpack has three stitched-in solar panels connected to a lithium battery that are sturdy enough to withstand rough treatment. It can be used to recharge portable electronic devices such as mobile phones. Users found one day's British spring sunshine provided sufficient energy to recharge a mobile phone.

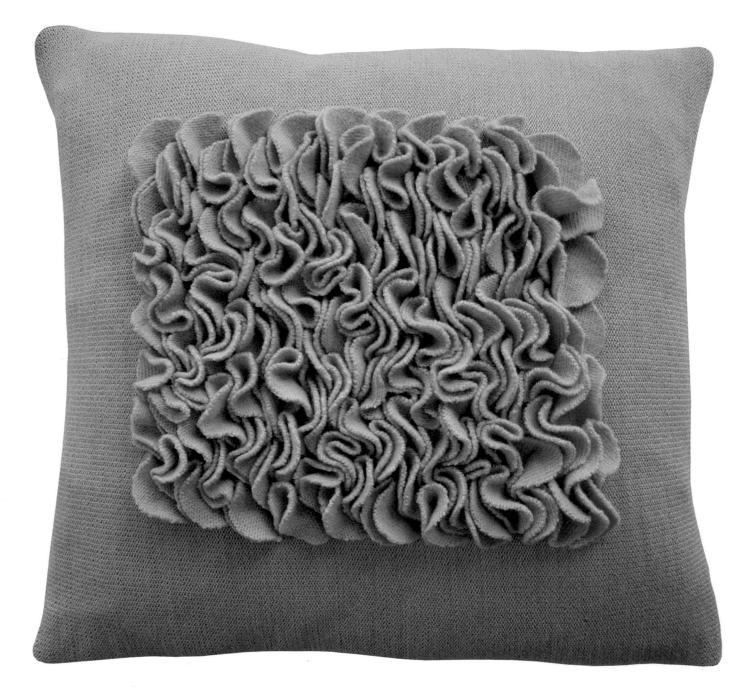

LoooLo, a Toronto-based company, develops textiles made from certified organic buckwheat and cotton, as well as Climatex Lifecycle yarns (organic fibres free of toxins and hazardous bio-products). Raw materials are grown mostly by local Canadian farmers, then dyed in a closed-loop facility, where remainders from the dye baths are purified, recycled and reused entirely, never releasing pollutants to the outside. Products no longer needed can be composted and will completely biodegrade and be reabsorbed into the earth within one year.

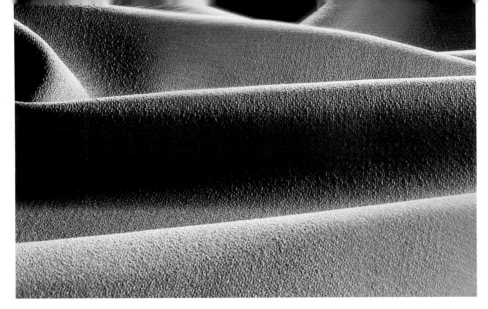

Climatex Lifecycle, 1995, manufactured by Rohner Textil AG (Switzerland) is made from ramie and wool. The entire textile production manufacturing process was ecologically revamped with the assistance of staff from the Environmental Protection Encouragement Agency. Considerable effort was made to test dyes for ecological safety. Although a mere 16 out of 1600 available dye chemicals lived up to the rigid specifications, the entire spectrum of colour was achieved except black. Climatex fabric is not only biodegradable, but also the waste material from weaving can be converted into felt to be used as non-wovens for upholstery work or as a mulch in the garden. The felt is ideally suited for the cultivation of strawberries, cucumbers and a wide range of other plants and is absolutely harmless to humans and the environment.

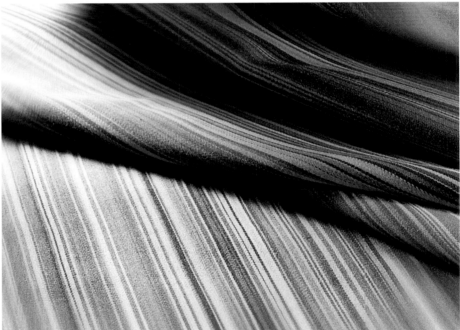

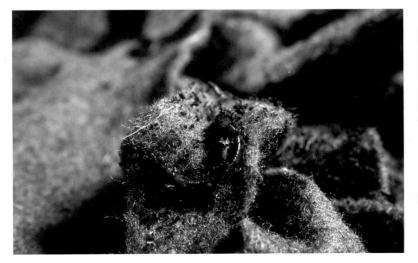

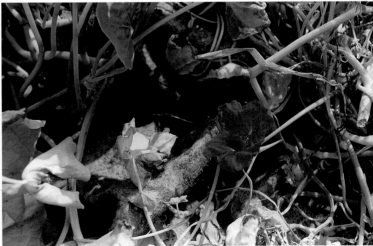

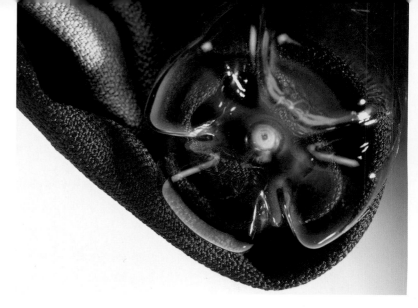

begun to be at least as concerned with where food has come from as with its appearance. These concerns mean that a more holistic approach to design – characterized by a shift from the conventional preoccupation with form and surface appearance to a broader concern with materials, systems and the consumption of energy – has started to be regarded as good design practice.

Faced with such complex issues a new, more collaborative approach to design has emerged which involves a chemical engineer and the designers sitting side by side. Two of the most successful pioneers of this approach are the American architect William McDonough and his collaborator the German chemical engineer and former Greenpeace activist Professor Michael Braungart. In the mid-1990s they developed a method of working that went beyond the traditional design brief to what they perceived to be the real problem that a designer should be tackling. Rather than concentrating exclusively upon a fabric's appearance, their model for developing 'ecologically intelligent' fabrics involved a re-assessment of all the materials and processes used in the system of fabric production and its supply chain. Dyestuffs, chemicals, bleaches and catalysts – as well as the suitability of the textile itself for recycling – came under their scrutiny in turn. Drawing an analogy between textiles and food there is a distinction between (1) biological

nutrients – disposable natural textiles where every component of textile manufacture feeds into natural cycles of growth and decay and (2) technical nutrients which can be recycled without a substantial decline in product quality and which feed into closed-loop systems of industrial production, thereby limiting the demand for dwindling fossil fuels. Nylon 6 can be used to make durable, recyclable carpets because it can be easily depolymerized into its precursor, caprolactam, that can in turn be repolymerized and remade into an even better version of Nylon 6. It is a good technical nutrient because its chemical composition is simple. By contrast Nylon 6.6, the far more famous version developed by Wallace Carothers' research team at DuPont in 1938, is comprised of two separate components which makes it impossible to recycle through depolymerization.

In addition, material awareness is being enhanced by digital culture. The internet is creating a demand for textile products that are made from materials that tell a story. Early pioneers such as the Swiss company Freitag Lab (who began making messenger bags from recycled truck tarpaulins in 1993) have now been joined by a host of other companies such as Modulab from Chile, Escama from Brazil and Vaho Works and Demano from Spain, who recycle promotional banners to make bags, clothing and footwear.

Interface Fabrics (USA), *Terratex*. Interface Fabrics is one of the biggest manufacturers of contract furnishings in the world. In 1995 they launched Terratex, one of the first commercial carpeting fabrics to be made from recycled, second-hand polyester fabrics and reclaimed wool. The range of recycled and compostable materials used in this range has now expanded to include plastic bottles and bio-based polymers. These are derived from crops rich in starch such as maize, sugarbeet or rice. The starch is converted into sugar and fermented to produce lactic acid which is then processed and polymerized. By 2003 they were purchasing sufficient wind energy to manufacture a million yards of Terratex cloth.

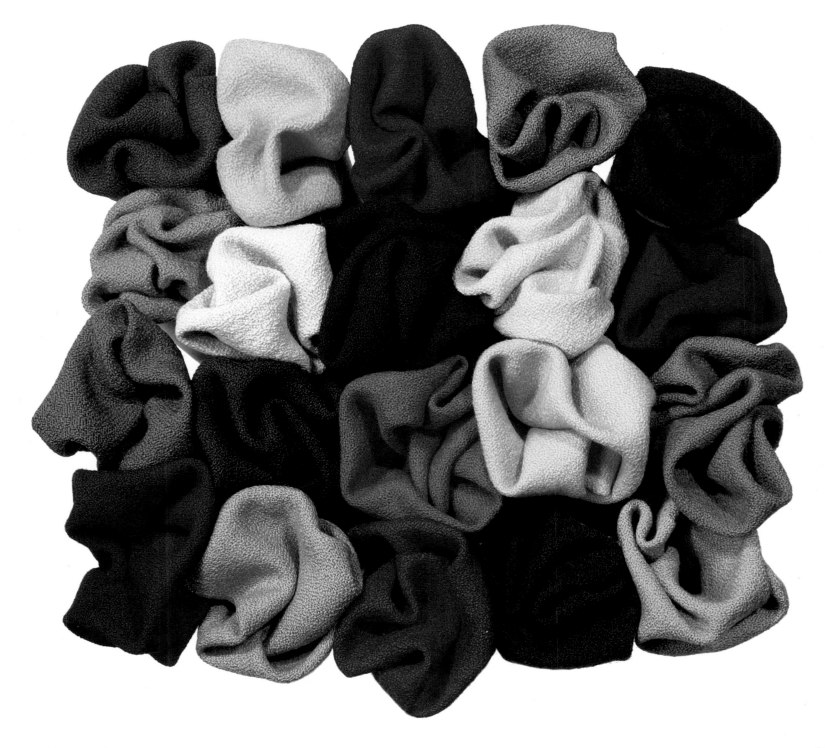

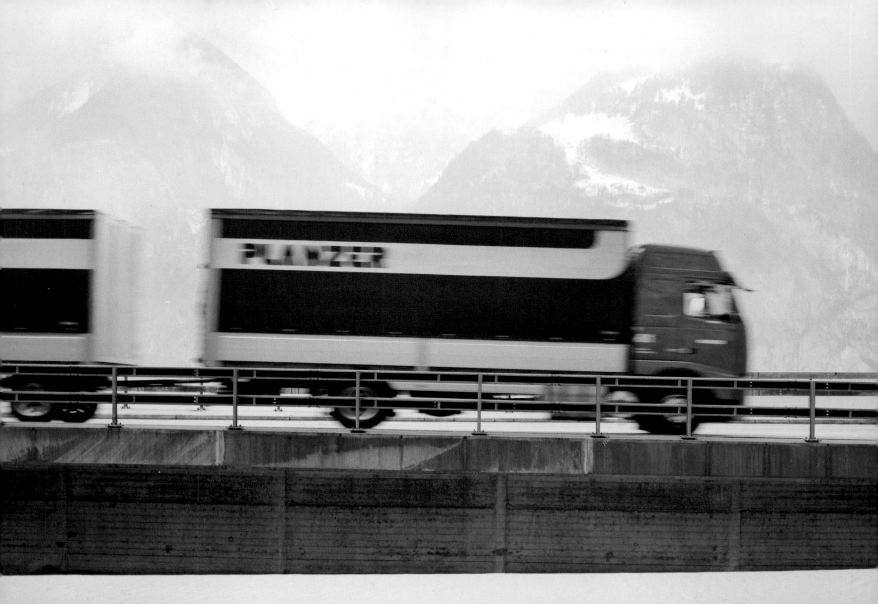

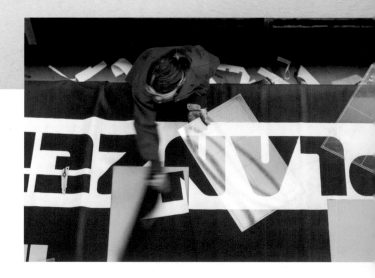

Freitag Lab AG (Switzerland) have turned recycling into an international business. Their messenger bags are entirely made from recycled materials such as used truck tarpaulins, bicycle innertubes, seatbelts and airbags. The bags are now distributed worldwide.

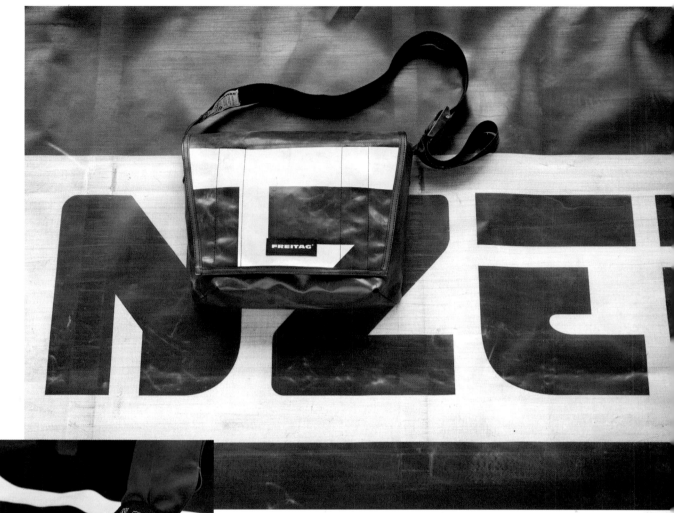

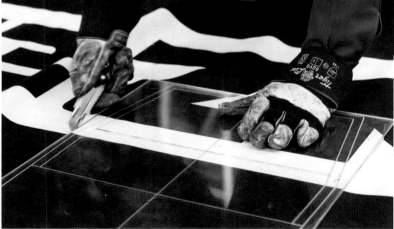

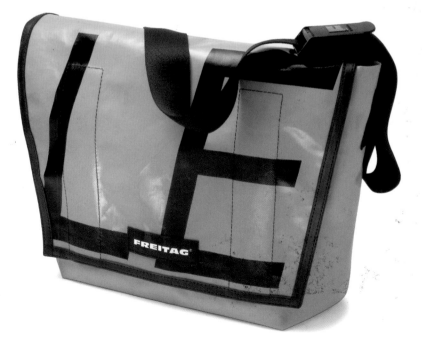

Demano (Spain), set up in 1999, uses promotional banners as the raw material to make a wide range of products including boots and bags.

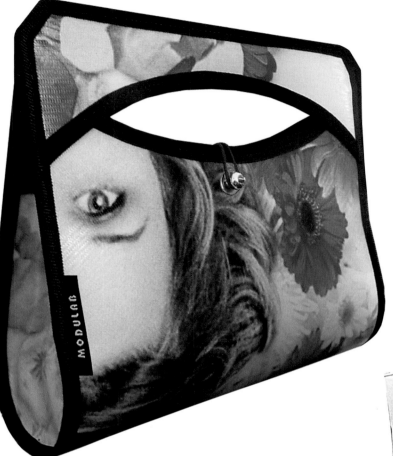

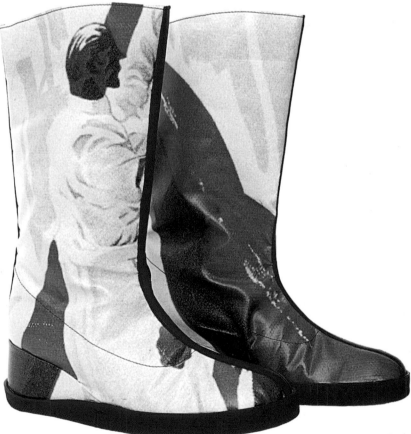

Modulab (Chile), 2005. Modulab is a design
studio that recycles advertising banners
to produce accessories such as bags and
wallets.

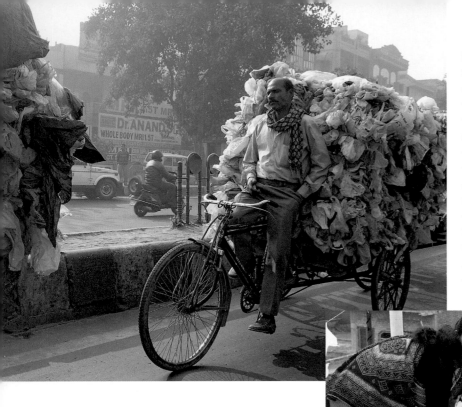

Bag made from recycled plastic by Conserve India, 2005. This bag is a remarkable example of a recycling and waste management scheme that has turned into a successful commercial enterprise. Conserve is a waste management NGO that was founded by Shalabh and Anita Ahuja in 2003 to address the mounting problem of domestic waste in the poorer areas of New Delhi. It converts a waste problem – polythene bags that block the drains and litter the streets – into fashionable hand bags and employs 60 women. Ragpickers are commissioned to gather and sort polythene bags. They are then washed, sorted by colour and moulded into thick, colourfully patterned plastic sheets by being passed through heated rollers. The colours you see are derived from the way the bags are arranged in the press. The sheets are cut and stitched into a range of tote bags and purses that are marketed internationally.

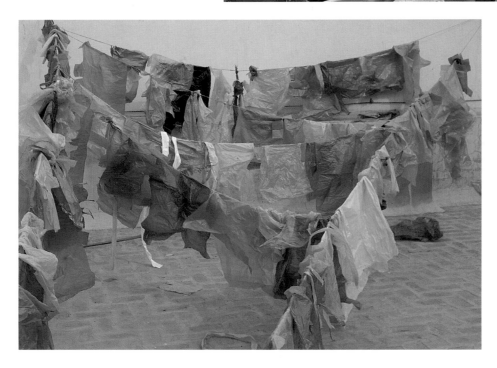

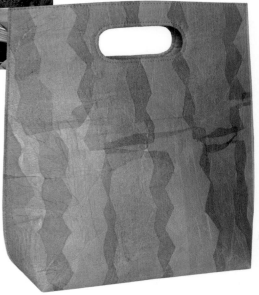

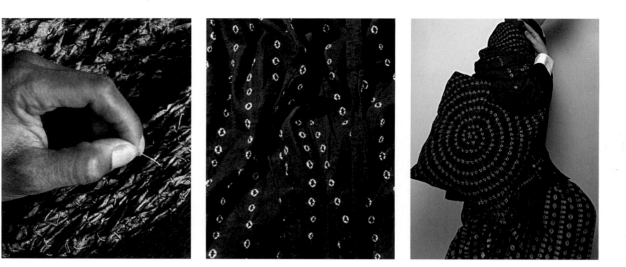

Heartwear is a non-profit organization that helps artisans in developing countries to tailor their products to the tastes of western consumers without compromising their skills and expertise or polluting their environment. The project was initially launched when Li Edelkoort visited Benin in the company of a group of stylists in 1993; it has since extended its activities to Morocco and India.

Conserve, a New Delhi non-governmental organization, which has recently grown out of a recycling and waste management project started by Shalabh and Anita Ahuja in 2003, is a good example of a local material recycling initiative that has successfully transferred to an international market through the tactical employment of foreign designers. They take moulded multi-coloured sheets of plastic made from recycled plastic bags collected and sorted by ragpickers in the slums of New Delhi and make sewn handbags that are available to a worldwide internet audience. Heartwear, launched by trend prediction analyst Li Edelkoort in 2003, is another example of this phenomenon. Here the aim is to safeguard existing craft practices in West Africa (and the livelihoods that depend on them) from being driven into obsolescence by foreign imports (such as European second-hand clothing) by developing them into products that are intended to sustain existing skills while being attractive to a foreign market.

Projects such as these indicate two important shifts: in terms of where traditional design skills are being applied and in terms of who is doing the designing. The projects show that to achieve socially or environmentally progressive outcomes designers must form part of a team. It is an approach to design that is fundamentally at odds with the culture of celebrity design which became prominent in the second half of the 20th century. In the case of Edelkoort's conservation project the role of the European designer takes a secondary role: their aim is to facilitate other people's creativity. In the case of Conserve, design is used to market and therefore fund a social waste management and social rehabilitation project. And with the textiles designed by the McDonough team the design of industrial process and material flows takes precedence over the surface design of the fabric.

These low-tech projects are encouraging consumers to think of textile materials as having a lifecycle, as if they were a plant or an animal and not just a man-made thing. If we apply this way of thinking to the sophisticated man-made materials that were developed for the textile industry in the first few years of the 21st century, the question that this raises is 'how well adapted are they to life over the longer term?', as Benyus puts it. Few of the dazzling, multi-functional fabrics described in the first sections of this chapter have been designed with recycling as a primary concern. Thus while nanotechnology is drawing inspiration from nature to bring about a revolution in thinking about the properties and surfaces, it is on these wider issues that scientists need to focus their attention now.

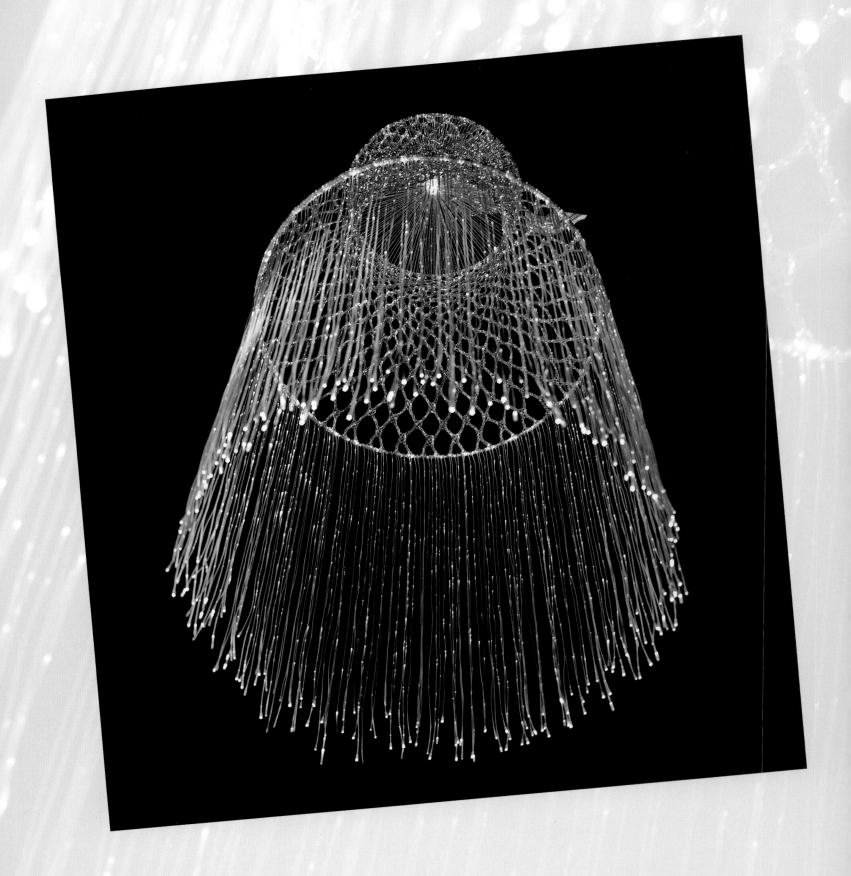

Objects

Over the past decade both designers and architects have begun to show an increased interest in textiles. Their interest encompasses two opposing tendencies. On the one hand, many designers and architects have been stimulated by the possibilities presented by new textile technologies and by textiles whose practical functions – to provide shadow, or comfort, or support, for example – are being reinvented by the incorporation of lighting or electronics. On the other hand, there has been a revival of interest in vintage fabrics, such as French linens, and local vernacular traditions, as well as craft textiles and popular crafts, such as knitting and crochet; all aspects of textile practice that have conventionally been excluded from, or which have developed in opposition to, classical modernist aesthetics.

In the first few years of the millennium the marriage between 1970s craft aesthetics, e-textiles and computing became a feature of interactive design. Yet this was also a period when designers began to work with metallicized fabrics and inflatables to create versatile fabric dwellings, shelters and transformable or multi-purpose objects. Designers were stimulated by the potential of new textile technologies and yet they also became interested in the inherent flexibility of fabric, its capacity to be folded and unfolded in different ways. Although such objects and structures showed how much designers remained influenced by modernist aspirations, they also revealed how complex designers' relationship to the modernist tradition had become.

Neils van Eijk (Dutch), *Bobbin Lace Lamp*, 2002. A lace lamp made from a 500-metre skein of fibre optic filament. When fibre optic filaments are forced to conform to conventional lace-making techniques their internal glass sheath snaps as it is knotted, allowing light to escape at these points, thereby making this lace lampshade into the light source.

Marcel Wanders (Dutch), *Knotted Chair*, 2001, already held to be an iconic example of turn of the millennium celebrity design because of the way it marries past and present and low-tech craft practice with high-tech materials. The chair is made from a composite aramid and carbon fibre rope, which is knotted using a macramé technique and then soaked in epoxy resin before being dried into shape by being suspended on a frame. It was originally made as part of the Droog Design collective's *Dry Tech* project, which was set up in 1995 in collaboration with the department of Space and Aviation at the University of Delft. The word droog means 'dry', as in 'dry wit', in Dutch, and the project aimed to show that even state-of-the-art materials could be made to tell a story. *Knotted Chair* has been acquired by the Museum of Modern Art in New York, a status that is reflected in its price. Over a thousand chairs have been made by hand at the Wanders Wonders workshop in Amsterdam, but as Wanders has admitted, 'photos of *Knotted Chair* are more important than the chair itself': during the past decade it has become known to millions through being reproduced in newspapers, magazines and books.

Bertjan Pot (Dutch), *Carbon Copy Chair*, 2003. Carbon fibre chair strengthened with epoxy resin. Modelled on Charles and Ray Eames' *DSR Chair* (1948). Manufactured by Wanders Wonders, Amsterdam.

For although the hypothetical future that some designers began to envisage remains one of technological innovation – in the sense that it is hoped that new textile technologies might enable people to learn to live with less – it was simultaneously implicitly critical of models of development based upon the idea of economic growth and increased productivity. More recently, state-of-the-art fabrics have been developed which aim to improve the living conditions of refugees and other people without access to basic amenities. Many of these projects have a utopian feel to them – at worst they are otherworldly and at best fabric technologies are being developed and adapted to suit local requirements and problems on the ground.

Knotted Chair (2001), made by the Dutch designer Marcel Wanders from rope impregnated with a polymer resin, is an iconic piece of 21st-century furniture design that achieves a synthesis of these oppositional tendencies discussed above. It integrates two seemingly incompatible elements: macramé (a craft redolent of the 1970s disillusionment with modernism and the technocratic vision of progress) with classic modernist office furniture design. It is an example of the way that the modernist tradition, which is clearly expressed in the new textile technologies that surround us today, is being adapted to suit contemporary sensibilities.

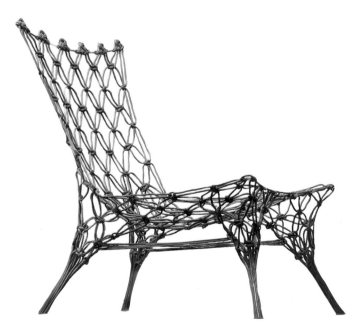

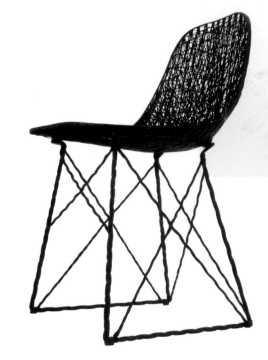

Marcel Wanders (Dutch), *Zeppelin*, 2005.
Chandeliers sprayed with cocoon resin,
manufactured by Flos, Italy. A reinterpretation of the classic Cocoon lighting
collection designed by Achille Castiglione
for Flos in 1962, when spraying fibre
glass had just become available on the
market; Wanders' chandeliers festooned in
fibre-glass cobwebs play on the correlation
between tradition and innovation.

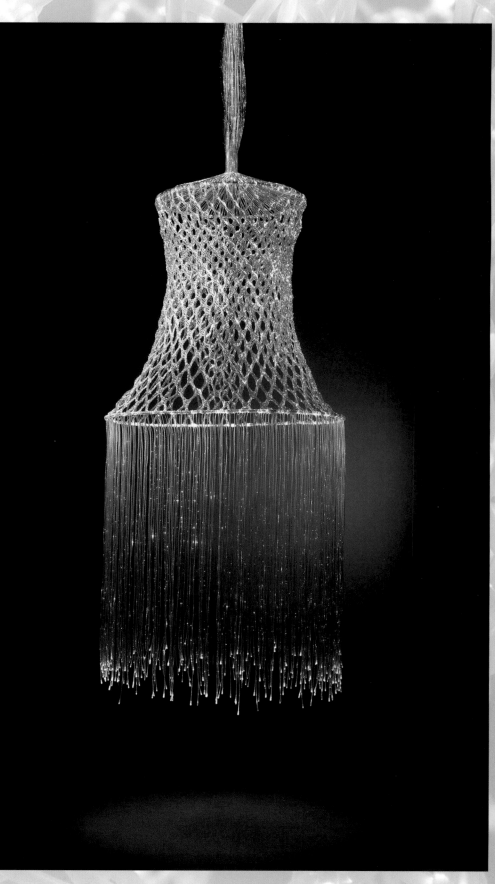

Neils van Eijk (Dutch), *Bobbin Lace Lamp*, 2002. The lampshade is made from 500 metres of fibre glass which is knotted using a bobbin lace technique.

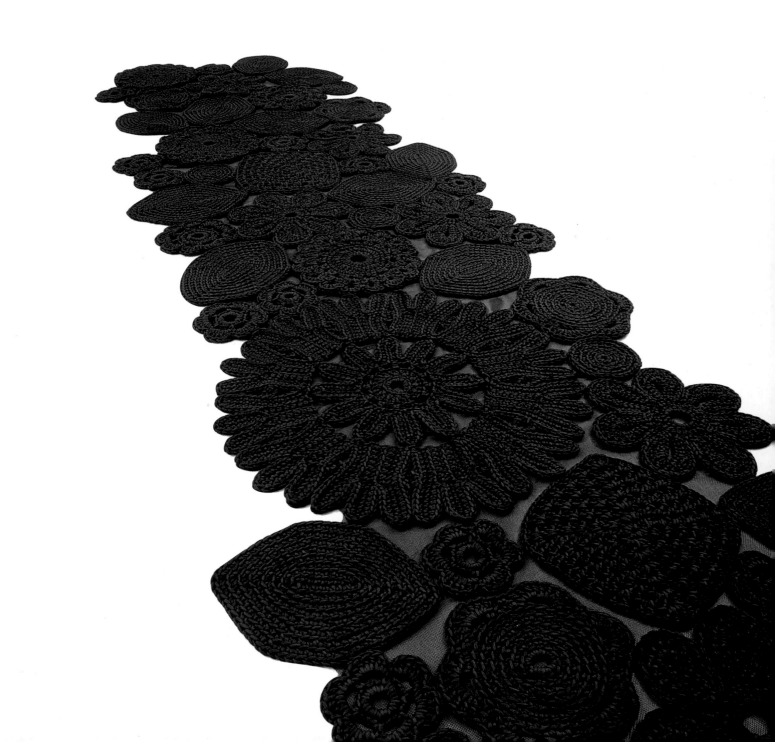

Paola Lenti (Italy), *Crochet Rug*, 2004. Hand-crocheted rug made from synthetic fibre.

Fabric Architecture

Towards the turn of the millennium architects, designers and artists began to use new textiles to create futuristic fabric shelters, dwellings and stadia. Architectural fabrics and membranes were used on a greater scale than ever before on public building projects. A single order from Saudi Arabia for The Mina Valley development for pilgrims to the Haj required a greater yardage of Teflon-coated cloth than German company Hightex had ever manufactured. In Britain as well fabrics and membranes began to be used on landmark public buildings such as the Millennium Dome in London and the Eden Project in Cornwall. In Germany and the United States architects started to envisage buildings that would largely be composed of fabric.

The lead up to the millennium was a time when policy makers and research institutes promoted a revival of a vision of the future determined by progress in science and new technology. With her *Refuge Wear* series (1992–98) British artist Lucy Orta re-interpreted the ultra-futuristic, space-age visions of a flexible, nomadic urban way of life (such as the futuristic hypothetical dwellings envisaged by the British architectural group Archigram with their *Plug-in-City* [1968] where the city was replaced by a framework into which dwellings in the form of cells could be slotted or the *Walking City* envisaged by Ron Herron [1964] where people dwelt in self-contained living pods subsequently developed by

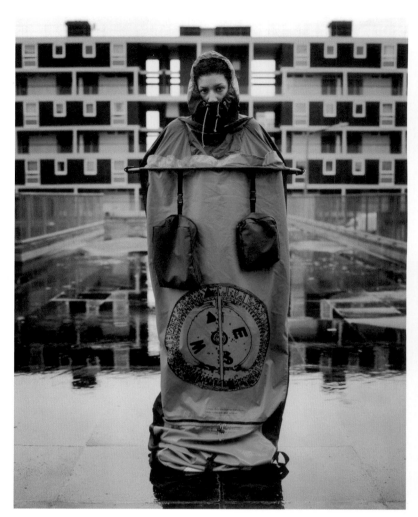

Archizoom, Superstudio and Future Systems) in the light of the contemporary reality of homelessness, displacement and alienation.

Experimental textile structures that explored the relationship between clothing and architecture such as Orta's *Habitent* (1992–93) made from aluminium coated, fleece-lined polyamide, or her adapted parkas, led people to question such technological optimism by translating the rudimentary dwellings made from sleeping bags and cardboard boxes of the homeless into the high-performance fabrics of the moment. An ongoing, related project, *Nexus Architecture* (begun in 1993), consisting of a collection of boiler suits linked together by a

Lucy Orta (UK), *Refuge Wear*, 1998, London. British artist Lucy Orta is widely held to have influenced the revival of interest in humanitarian design and in making fabric shelters for refugees and the homeless in the late 1990s. Her approach was to make symbolic clothing – dwellings that would attract media attention about the plight of the homeless. Over the years designers inspired by her work have begun to move away from her emphasis on symbolism to take a more pragmatic approach to these issues.

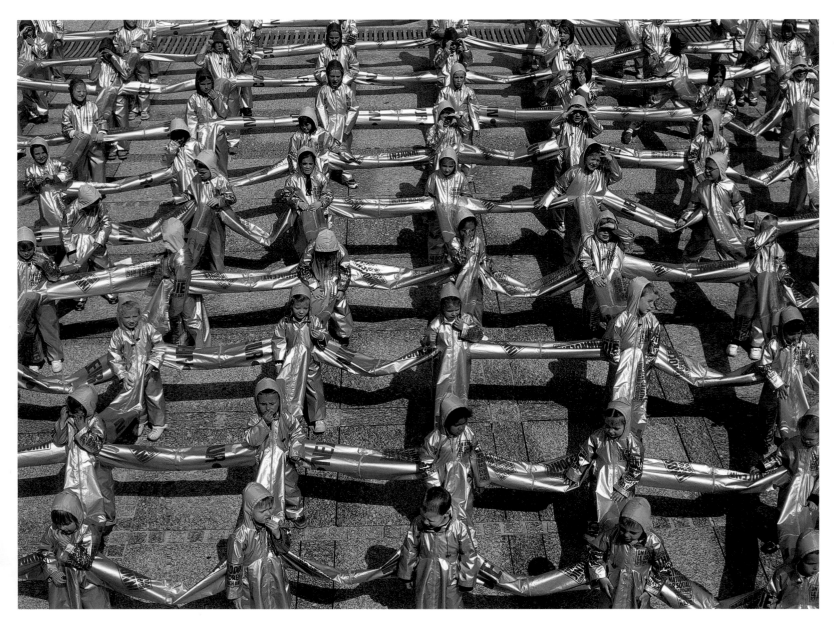

network of fabric tubes and zippers, was worn by participants to mount public protests against a range of issues such as child labour and the Rwanda Genocide, in demonstrations that created a social sculpture. Orta's *Refuge Wear* revived interest in transformables – versatile pieces of clothing that could be turned into shelters or rudimentary pieces of furniture. CP Company, the Italian menswear producer, developed a line of inflatable clothes. These garments were packaged with an air compressor that could be plugged into a car's lighter, enabling them to assume the form of blow up armchairs, mattress-tent combinations and so on.

Lucy Orta (UK), *Nexus Wear*, 2001. This work exploits the symbolism of modernist clothing to raise questions about the impact of modernist ideas of progress upon the environment and social wellbeing. Performers dressed in outfits that superficially resemble spacesuits or the kind of protective overalls used by Greenpeace activists are linked to each other by 'umbilical' fabric tubes connected by zippers. Different variations of this fabric architecture have been performed by adults and children in several contexts and settings, including Cologne Cathedral, Germany, the Global March against Child Labour and the 2nd Johannesburg Biennale, South Africa.

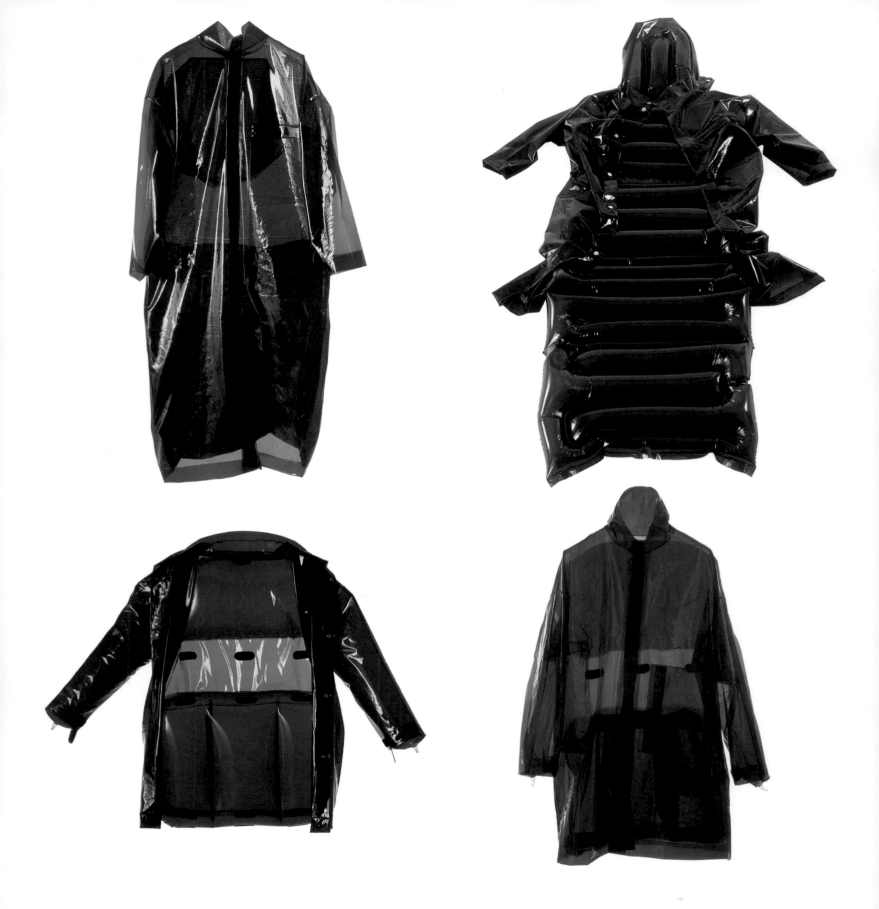

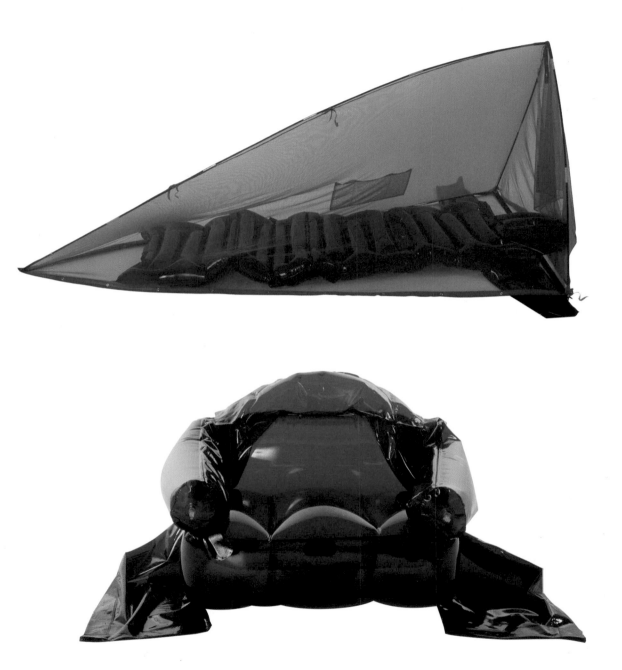

Moreno Ferrari (Italy), *Parka – Armchair* from the *Transformables Collection*, 2001 (opposite). Polyurethane sections of this parka coat have been inflated to form a blow-up chair.

Parka – Air-Mattress from the *Transformables Collection*, 2001 (above). All manufactured by CP Company, Bologna.

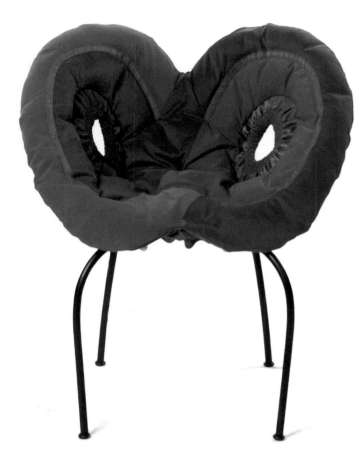

In a related project, Japanese architect and expert computer programmer, Dai Fujiwara, began to collaborate with the celebrated Japanese fashion designer Issey Miyake. Called *A-Poc* (short for 'a piece of cloth'), this project (begun in 1997) involved the use of an industrial knitting or weaving machine that had been programmed by a computer. The resultant tubes of fabric were assembled in such a way that both the garment form and pattern were integral to the fabric itself – all the consumer had to do was to cut the pieces free from the cloth.

Catalan designer Martín Ruiz de Azúa's interest in textile shelters is driven by his belief that we are destined to live with less. Textile technologies, Azúa believes, may provide the key for consumer culture to redeem itself. Living with less will soon be possible, he suggests, because technology will enhance the performance of materials to such an extent that many of the objects that currently encumber us and our homes will simply disappear, as they are absorbed into fewer, more versatile products.

Basic House (1999) is a house of air which conveys an extreme vision of the future – of buildings that materialize and vanish when they are no longer needed and of cities where people live like modern nomads in inflatable houses that fold up and travel with them wherever they go. Made from double-sided metallicized polyester, Azúa's

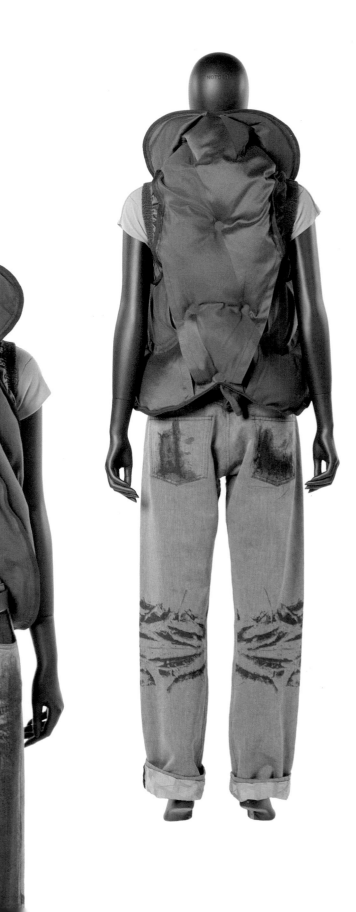

Dai Fujiwara (Japan), *Trampoline and Gemini*, 2006. Made by the Miyake Design Studio.

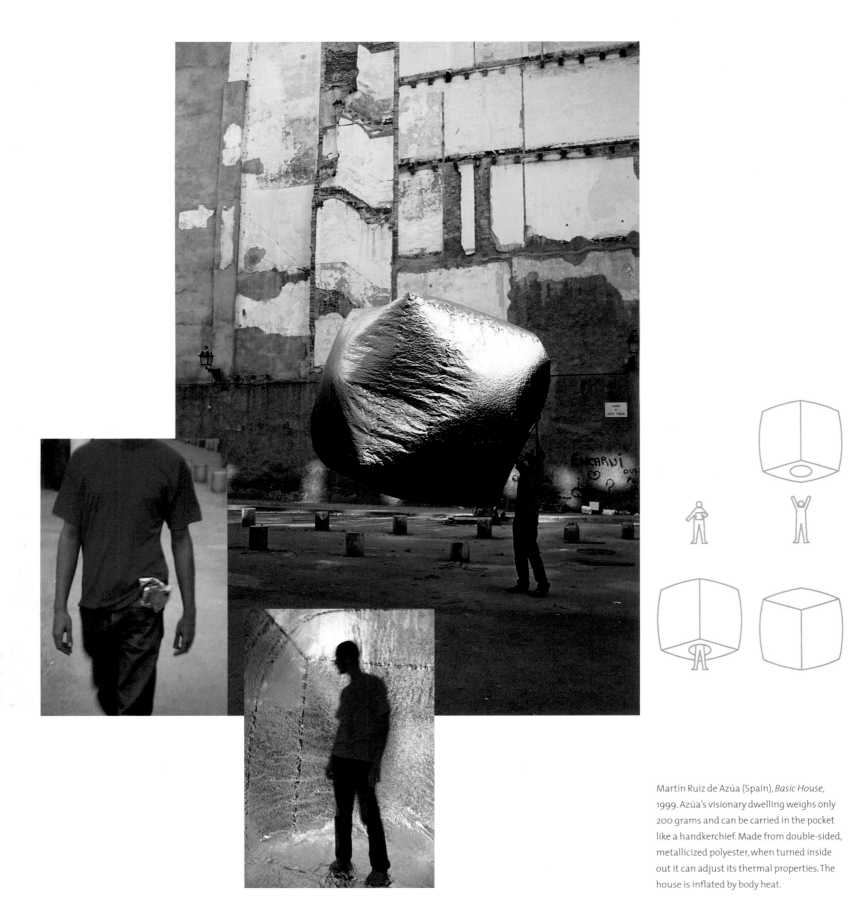

Martín Ruiz de Azúa (Spain), *Basic House*, 1999. Azúa's visionary dwelling weighs only 200 grams and can be carried in the pocket like a handkerchief. Made from double-sided, metallicized polyester, when turned inside out it can adjust its thermal properties. The house is inflated by body heat.

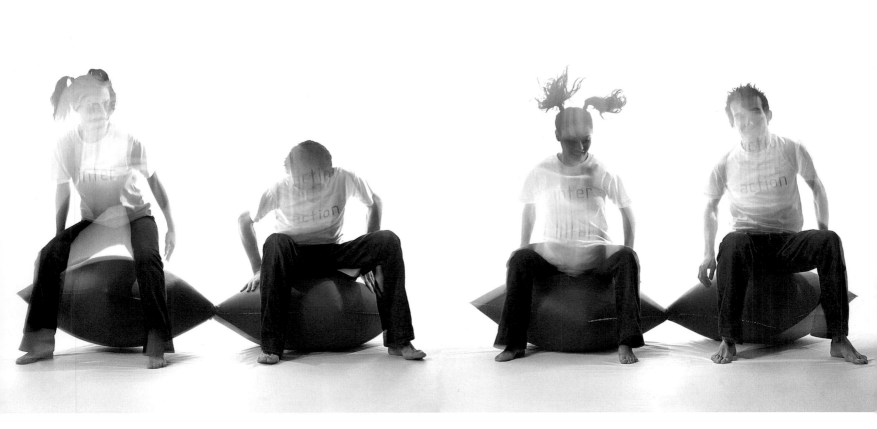

Martín Ruiz de Azúa (Spain), *Interactive Cushion*, 2000. Two interconnecting inflated cushions made from plastic communicate movement between the users.

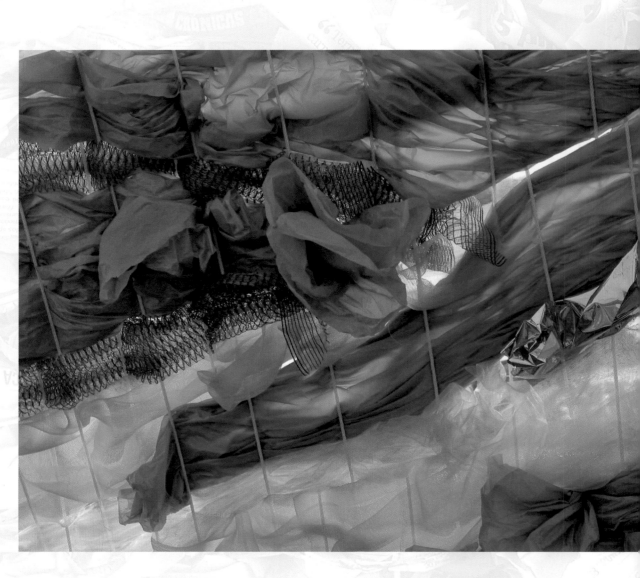

Martín Ruiz de Azúa (Spain), *Valla/Plaited
Fence*, 2003. A curved partition simply made
of a series of galvanized steel frames is
mounted with a string warp (detail, above),
creating a lattice into which a range of
recycled materials can easily be woven.

'house in a pocket' weighs only 200 grams and can be inflated by the heat of the sun, or simply by the heat of one's body. It is silver on one side and gold on the other and can be reversed to offer protection from either the heat or the cold.

Work like this is, of course, visionary and utopian and does not pretend to offer practical solutions to existing problems. Azúa himself admits as much, saying that *Basic House* was made in response to the soaring price of property in Barcelona. Yet it is interesting to see where concept design can lead. In Azúa's case it has led to a length of traditional Catalan fabric that was once used to make the classic *Bossa Catalana* or 'Catalan Bundle', an item formerly employed by agricultural labourers to carry wood and food, or as a table cloth, but which could also provide shelter from the elements, if necessary. Azúa's version, developed in 2004, is being reproduced with the aid of a social rehabilitation initiative that involves an association of Catalan prison inmates. An artefact that synthesizes his interest in multi-purpose objects, sustainable design, social welfare and neo-rural vernacular, *Bossa Catalana* is a reminder that multi-purpose textile objects are not new, but are in fact a common feature of much traditional dress.

Could this suggest an approach towards 21st-century dress reform? Fashion has tended to pull in the opposite direction – that is, towards the increasingly complex differentiation of clothing in terms its style, fabric, cut and size (with greater emphasis on style and fabric for women's clothing and a greater accent on cut and size for menswear). Differentiations have tended to circumscribe the use of clothing, by limiting the range of occasions on which a garment can be worn or by curtailing the period of its use, and lie behind our unsustainable consumption of clothes.

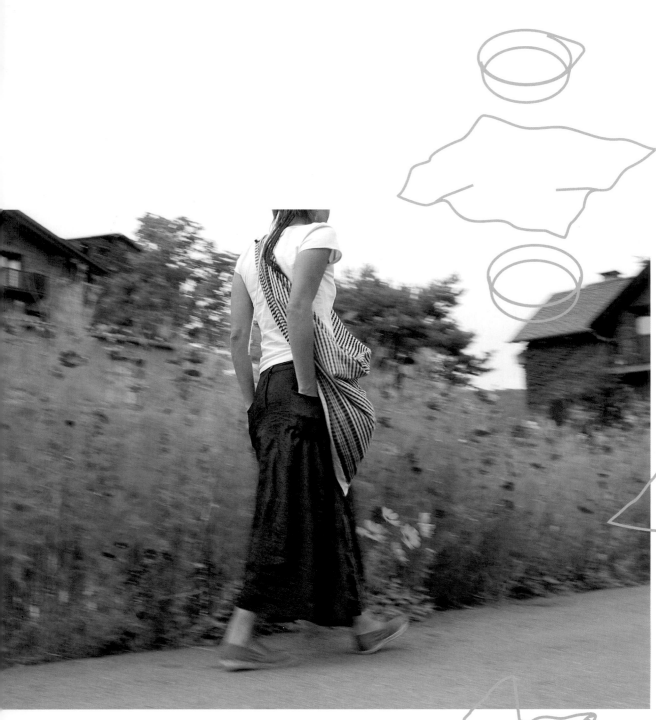
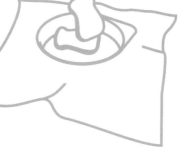

Martín Ruiz de Azúa (Spain), *Catalan Bag*, 2004. Made from the chequered cloth that traditionally served Catalan men working on the land as a bundle, table cloth, or shelter. It is an example of the way that environmental concerns are reviving interest in a more versatile approach to cloth. These bags are made with the aid of the Centre for Reinsertion Initiatives (CIRE) which co-ordinates workshops in Catalan prisons.

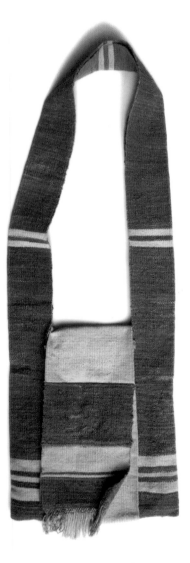
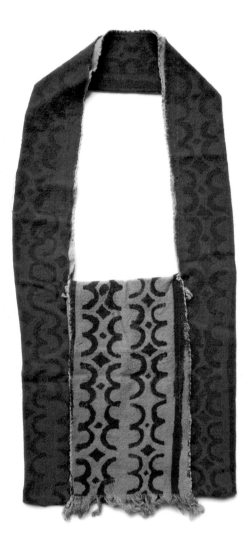
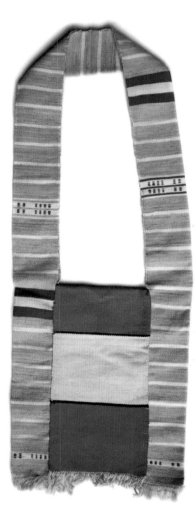

Anthony Labouriaux (France), *Woven Bag*. 1999. Developed in collaboration with strip weavers from Koho in Burkina Faso. While many approaches to sustainable design involve the transfer of new materials and technologies from the rich nations of the north to developing countries in the south, Labouriaux takes a different approach to sustainability by looking at how the local ways of making objects can be harnessed to help people sustain their livelihoods. This range of woven bags was developed for sale at the local market in Boromo where they continue to be a runaway success.

Azúa is not alone in thinking that new textile technologies and the tools and ideas for building a better future are close at hand. Sponsored by the European Space Agency Technology Transfer Programme, Italian architect Arturo Vittori of Architecture and Vision has created an experimental inflatable tent intended for use in extreme desert conditions. Like Azúa's *Basic House*, *Desert Seal* (2005) is supported by air, in this case inflatable airbeams. The tent is cooled by its fabric (a polyurethane-coated polyester), by a vent at the top of the tent which allows the passage of air and by a fan powered by newly developed solar film. It weighs 5.5 kg.

'Modern Nomad' is an example of reification: it shows how an idea such as 'population mobility' is changed into a cultural image that in turn inspires the design of objects. The virtue of such generalizations is that they can encompass a range of concerns; the danger is that an idea like this can take on a life of its own and become detached from real needs. Is progress inevitably associated with mobility? Some designers do not think so. Dutch tentmaker Dré Wapenaar's *Tree Tents (Boomtenten)* (1998) are made from conventional fabric. They were originally intended to shelter the Road Alert Group, an English association of environmental protestors who campaign to prevent road building through valued natural habitats, but the tents are now leased to holidaymakers.

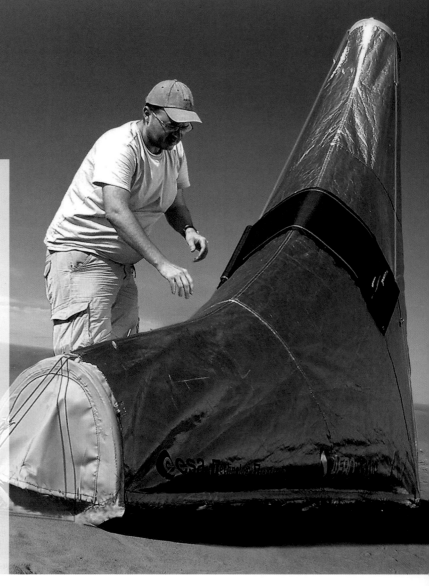

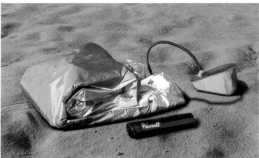

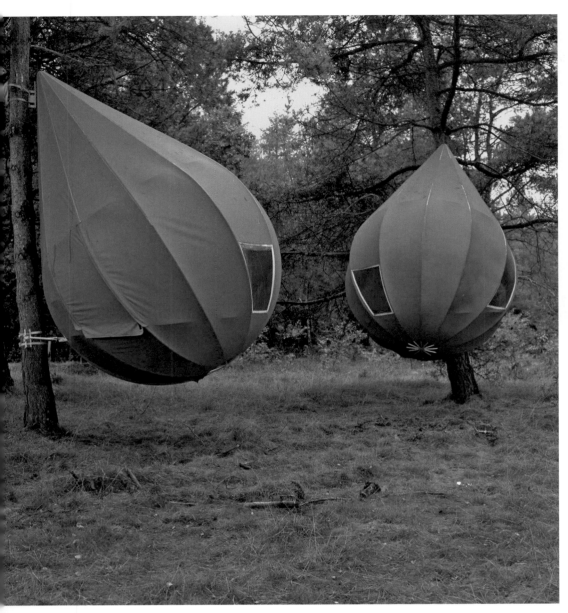

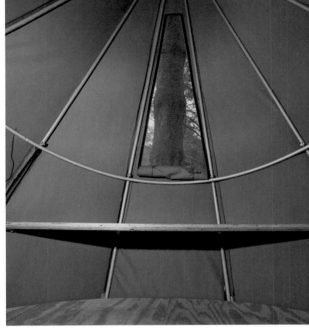

Dré Wapenaar (Dutch), *Tree Tents (Boomtenten)*, 1998. These tree tents have steel frames and are made of canvas with a wooden floor.

Arturo Vittori (Italy), *Desert Seal*, 2005 (opposite). An inflatable tent that exploits the temperature curve found in hot, arid regions. The curved shape allows the tent to be ventilated by cooler air which is taken as far as possible from the surface of the ground. Cooling is also enhanced by electric fans powered and by a band of flexible solar film on the tent's surface. The tent is made from polyethylene-coated polyester and is equipped with a silver-coated canvas awning to reflect as much heat as possible. The project is characteristic of the way that ecological concerns are encouraging designers to think about the interrelationship between buildings and the environment. This experimental prototype was developed in collaboration with the European Space Agency as part of their technology transfer programme.

More recent initiatives inspired by the idea of contemporary nomadic shelter adopt a research-based approach to design. An example is American architect Sheila Kennedy's *Portable Light Project* (2005), which was conducted under the 'Nomads and Nanomaterials Research Programme' at the department of architecture at the University of Michigan; it has now transferred to Harvard University.

According to current estimates, more than 2 billion people world-wide are without access to electricity, either because they live in remote rural areas, or because they live in regions affected by natural disaster or war. The *Portable Light Project* aimed to develop a series of proto-types for a portable, cost-effective textile light that would incorporate state-of-the-art solar cells and high-brightness light-emitting diodes, or HBLEDS, which could be useful in these situations. Even in small amounts, 'digital light' can help to improve educational opportunities, promote health and increase business opportunities. In consultation with members of the semi-nomadic Huichol (Wirrárica) community from the Mexican Sierra Madre, whose textiles continue to develop the tradition of Mesoamerican weaving, Kennedy developed a series of experimental textile lights and bags, again, in conjunction with a research group of architectural students at the University of Michigan.

Will Crawford and Peter Brewin (UK), *Concrete Canvas*, 2005. Cement-impregnated fabric has been bonded to the surface of an inflatable plastic lining. Regarded as a major innovation in the design of disaster shelters, Crawford Brewin's prototype emergency shelter was developed after they visited six different camps of internally displaced persons and after extensive consultation with UN agencies and various NGOs. It can be transported rapidly to the field of disaster, like a tent, and yet offers the improved shelter of a solid building. It can be used to protect medical equipment and stores and could also provide shelter for emergency relief workers or for displaced persons in danger of death from exposure.

Delivered folded and sealed in a sterile plastic sack weighing 230 kg, concrete canvas is light enough to be transported in the back of a pick-up truck or light aircraft and can be assembled by untrained personnel in 40 minutes. Once in position, the sack is filled with water. The tent is then unfolded and inflated with gas using a chemical activator. The concrete cloth curves, following the shape of the inflated lining and is ready to use within 12 hours. It is 16m sq and has a ten-year life span, which compares favourably with the two-year life span of conventional tents. Because it has a compressive structure it can be covered with earth and snow for insulation or can be covered with sandbags to protect against shrapnel.

Every component of the design has been optimized: the bag serves to reinforce the groundsheet, the canvas helps to wick water into the cement and improves the building's strength, and the building has been shaped so that it can serve agricultural purposes if it is no longer needed for emergency relief.

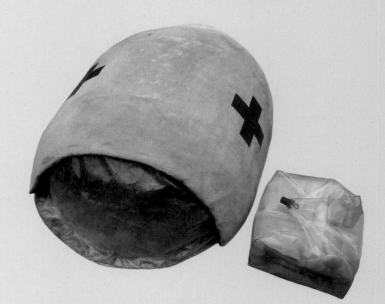

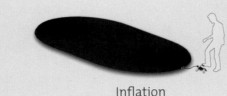
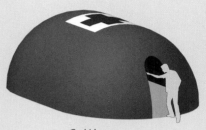

Delivery   Hydration   Inflation   Setting

Textiles were specifically chosen as the culturally appropriate medium for introducing new technologies, but it seems probable that the transformable garments discussed above would have also influenced the evolution of these prototypes. Their energy-harvesting backpacks can be unfolded and assembled into well-lit workshops, community shelters and portable lights during hours of darkness (roughly four hours charging time will provide 2 1/2 hours of digital light at 480 lumens). This project shows us how new textile technologies might be of service in real life situations. The *Community Bag*, for example, can seat six and could be useful for boosting trades such as *tortillerias*, bakeries and repair workshops at community gatherings. They are currently refining these prototypes through consultation with the Rocky Mountain Institute, a US non-profit organization that promotes efficient resource handling and will be distributing refined prototypes for a more extended period of field tests next year.

Young British designers Will Crawford and Peter Brewin have also developed a prototype tent that shows how experimental textile shelters can be developed through a research-based approach to design. Their interest in blow-up buildings was originally inspired by the use of inflatables as gas containers in industrial engineering. They wanted to see how a version of this fabric technology might serve some practical purpose for the 35 million refugees worldwide. They conducted three months fieldwork in Uganda with the United Nations High Commission for Refugees which included field trips to northern Uganda where a rebel paramilitary army had long been active. They then conducted over a hundred interviews with UN agencies and NGOs. This highlighted existing problems with tents securing medical equipment, insulation and durability (in Pakistan, tents were having to be replaced due to wind damage every three weeks). But the interviews also revealed problems with portable buildings, which were difficult to transport and slow to deploy, meaning that humanitarian agencies were often delayed in offering immediate relief in the event of a crisis.

Crawford and Brewin's shelter, made from cement-impregnated fabric, can be erected by an untrained person in 40 minutes and is ready to use in 12 hours, allowing humanitarian agencies to erect a building on the first day of arrival. By adding water to the bag and inflating it, this impregnated canvas sets in 4 hours and creates a hard emergency shelter. It can be delivered sterile, allowing a wide range of surgical operations to be performed in *situ*, can be made secure to protect medicine and equipment and can be insulated by adding sandbags.

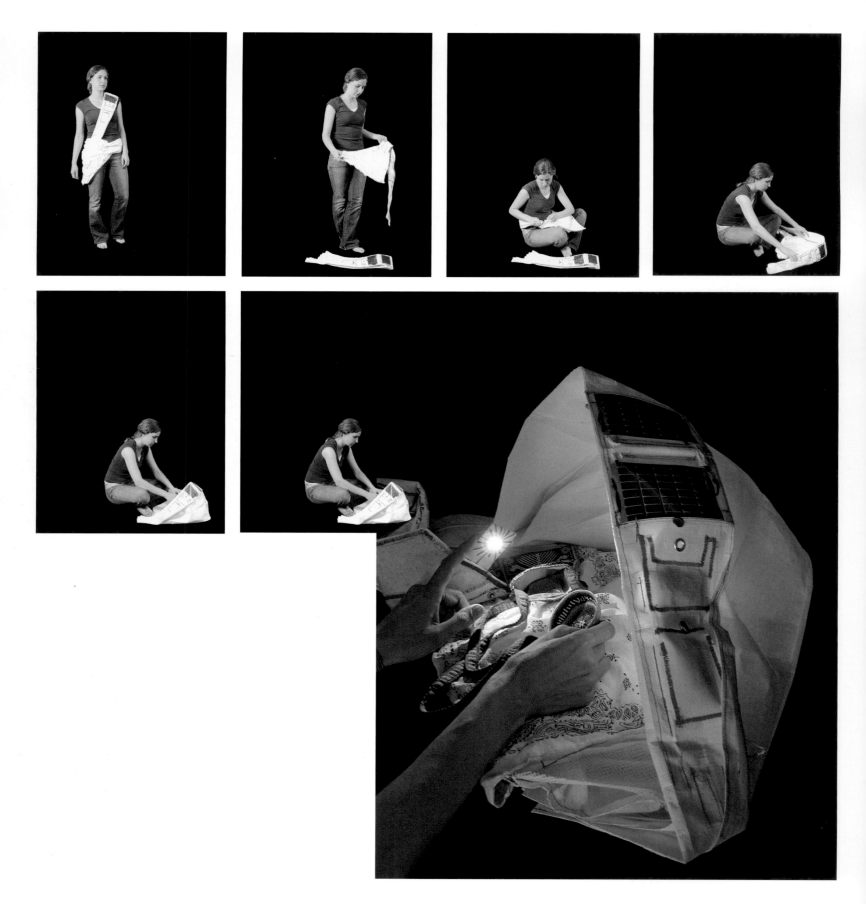

Sheila Kennedy (USA), *Community Bag* (opposite) and *Portable Mat* (below) from the *Portable Light Project*, 2005. The project offers series of adaptable, solar-powered fabric lights. The prototypes featured here were developed by Kennedy + Violich Architecture and the 'Nomads and Nanomaterials Research Programme' at the University of Michigan in consultation with advisors from the nomadic Huichol (Wirrárica) community who live in the Mexican Sierra Madre mountains. The idea was to create a series of light, wearable garments, such as sashes and backpacks, that could be unfolded to create workshops, small community tents, reading and cooking lights. Thin film solar cell panels charge polymer batteries which in turn power tiny, high brightness, light-emitting diodes that are embedded in a transluscent ripstop material. The result is a wearable, completely self-contained, off-the-grid solar-powered lighting system.

The prototypes are part of an initiative to provide lighting solutions for refugees and other people who lack access to electricity from a grid. The project is now undergoing a second phase of development in association with the Rocky Mountain Institute in Colorado, which specializes in sustainable design, and with students from the architectural department at Harvard University.

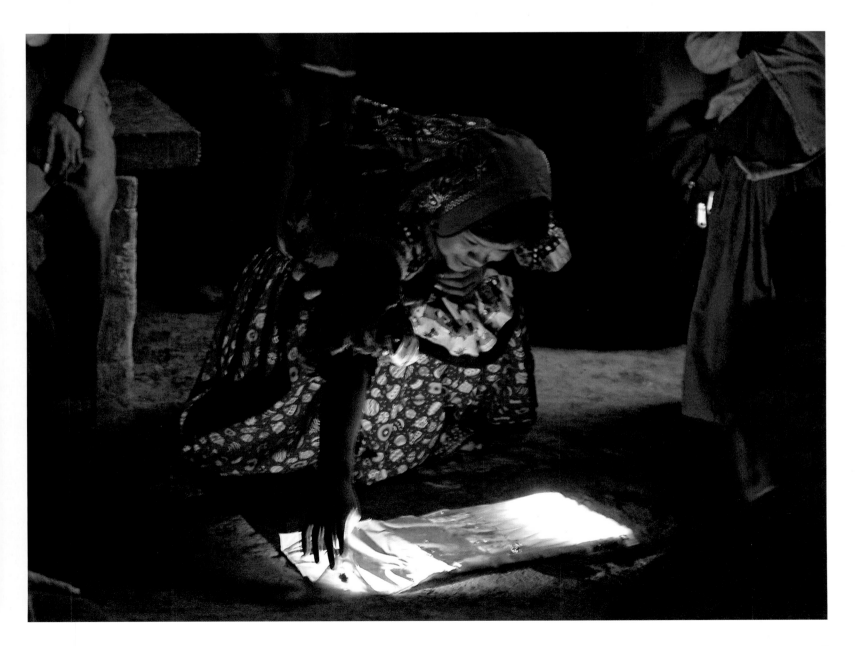

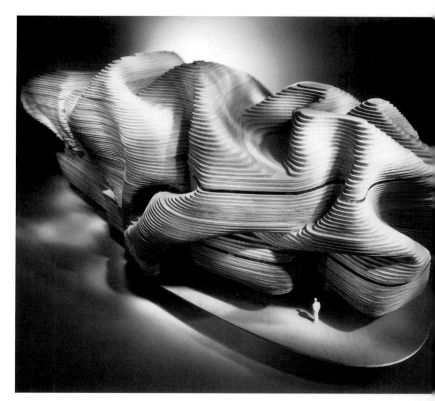

Architecture as Clothing

Seeing architecture as clothing presumes a distinction between the structural components of a building and its surface. It is a distinction that goes back to the inception of modernist architecture when, with the advent of steel frame construction (first developed in Chicago during the 1880s), walls lost their load-bearing function. Once the surface of the building became independent of a building's structure, walls could be seen as a covering that hung off the structural skeleton of the building, like a curtain, or a dress. Architecture became modernized through this new way of working at the surface of the building. Not only did many turn-of-the-century Viennese and German modernist architects experiment with dress design, but they also used the arguments of dress reform to strip away the classical or gothic garb worn by 19th-century buildings. Yet modernist buildings were not naked; architects envisaged that their athletic new buildings would be dressed in modern clothing inspired by the growing interest in sport.

However, it was the very proximity to fashion that prompted many modernist architects to distance themselves from it. Instead a new idiom for surface architecture was sought through examining the origins of architecture in tented structures, influenced by Gottfried Semper's 19th-century theories concerning the development of walls from earlier textile partitions and tented structures. Such scruples do not appear to be an issue today. The surface of a building is now discussed using the language of sportswear. It is perceived as a technical analogue for human skin that regulates the transmission of light, heat, moisture and other environmental pollutants. High-tech textiles and ETFE (ethylene tetrafluoroethylene) membranes have been used to recall futuristic structures envisaged by Jules Verne and Buckminster Fuller. With the construction of a series of iconic membrane structures – exhibition centres (the Eden Project, Cornwall, 2000 and the Millennium Dome, London, 2001) and stadia (the Allianz Arena in Munich, 2005 and the forthcoming Water Cube in Beijing, 2008), fabric architecture has reasserted itself at the start of the 21st century.

A good example of the renewed athleticism of architecture using contemporary textile technology is the experimental exhibition centre in Esslingen for the German pneumatic experts Festo AG and Co., developed in 2002 by their then head of corporate design, Axel Thallemer.

Thomas Heatherwick (UK) was commissioned by a Buddhist priest to design a new temple for the Shingon-Shu sect at Kagoshima, southern Japan, in 2005. To develop the design he scanned the folds of a thick piece of felt using the laser-scanning machine of a neighbouring hospital. Wrapping in fabric is a core feature of Japanese material culture and also an important aspect of Buddhist ritual. The completed building will be made of layers of glass and wood shaped in such a way as to resemble the undulating folds of this piece of cloth.

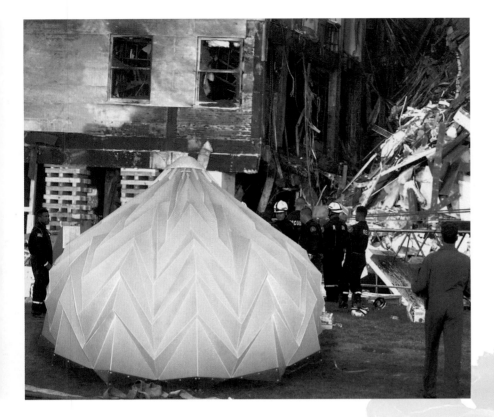

Jörg Student (Germany), *Ha-Ori Emergency Shelter*, 2004. Made of polypropolene, this prototype for an emergency shelter was modelled on the folds of a hornbeam leaf. The Ha-Ori (Japanese for 'folding leaf') shelter is constructed from corrugated polypropolene that has been folded in a series of trapezoidal shapes to create a rigid structure. When open, the shelter has a diameter of 3.8 m and a height of 2.6 m. When folded, the Ha-Ori measures 2.7 m x 0.5 m for easy transport.

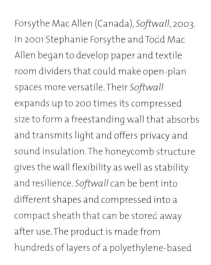

Forsythe Mac Allen (Canada), *Softwall*, 2003. In 2001 Stephanie Forsythe and Todd Mac Allen began to develop paper and textile room dividers that could make open-plan spaces more versatile. Their *Softwall* expands up to 200 times its compressed size to form a freestanding wall that absorbs and transmits light and offers privacy and sound insulation. The honeycomb structure gives the wall flexibility as well as stability and resilience. *Softwall* can be bent into different shapes and compressed into a compact sheath that can be stored away after use. The product is made from hundreds of layers of a polyethylene-based sheet material and is bounded by felt ends that serve as handles to adjust the wall's position and form a protective cover when the wall is folded for storage. The design is modular: the felt ends have Velcro strips that can link walls together. Manufactured by Molo Design, Vancouver.

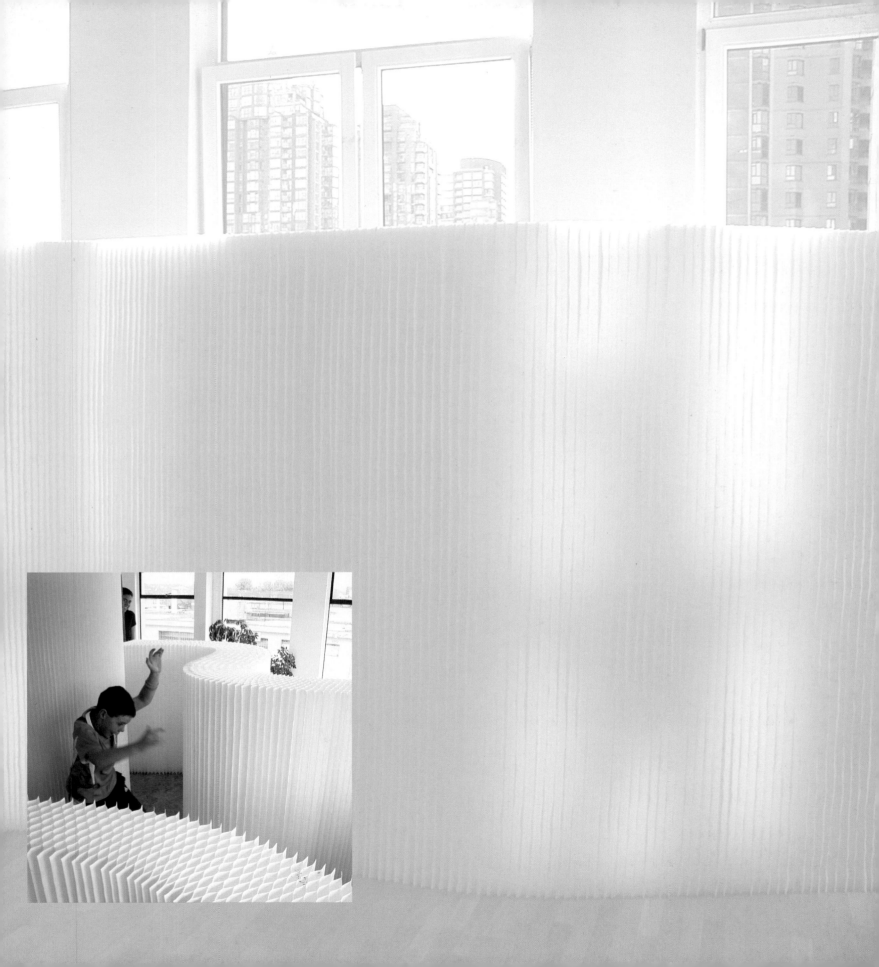

Axel Thallemer (Germany), *Airtecture*, 2001. The exhibition centre for Festo AG and Co., the German power tool and pneumatics firm. It is an inflatable building that demonstrates a new way of using textiles to harness the power of air. Unlike other recent membrane constructions that depend upon steel frames or cabling, Thallemer's *Airtecture* uses membranes and pressurized air as load-bearing materials. Inflated Y-shaped flying buttresses, inspired by the Y-shaped joints of dragonflies' wings, as much as by Gothic architecture, are held in dynamic tension by artificial textile muscles.

Axel Thallemer (Germany), *Fluidic Muscle*. Won Japan's Good Design Award in 1998 and is a hose consisting of alternating layers of elastomer and high-tensile fibres such as M5 and Kevlar that can contract and stretch like a muscle. It works with compressible fluids (such as air) as well as with non-compressible fluids (such as water).

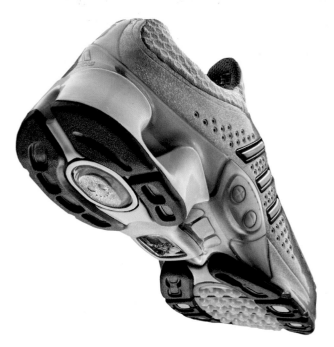

Adidas_1, launched in 2005. This shoe provides intelligent cushioning by automatically and continuously adjusting itself. The system works like an artificial muscle. A computerized magnetic sensing system is used to activate a motorized cable that pulls on the plastic cushioning, varying its softness.

This is a building that seems to be literally flexing its muscles. The aim was to construct a building entirely of fabric, where even the load-bearing structure would be made of inflated textile components. Y-shaped flying buttresses, whose form is inspired by the structure of a dragonfly's wing, hold the building in dynamic tension with the help of fluidic muscles, hoses comprised of alternating layers of elastomer and fibres that can be used as an actuator (i.e., a textile muscle connected to a computer). The result is a textile structure that changes according to the ambient conditions of sun, wind, rain or snow. Three computers read the ambient wind speed and temperature, flexing the pneumatic muscles as needed to keep the walls taut and erect, bleeding air from the roof when it grows warm and begins to expand. The interior is spanned by an inflatable roof, which is indented by a vacuum that keeps it taut. The windows themselves consist of four membranes. What distinguishes this building from previous air-supported structures is the use of much higher air pressure to create load-bearing structures that are stable enough to withstand the effect of southern German gales with windspeeds of up to 50 miles per hour (80 km/h) and in winter, the accumulation of snow on the roof.

The idea that architectural textiles can facilitate a dynamic relationship between the internal and external environment of a building has been developed in a variety of ways. With the Allianz Arena in Munich, completed in 2005, Swiss architects Jacques Herzog and Pierre de Meuron have created a sports stadium that can change its football strip. Capable of holding 69,901 people, it is the largest ETFE membrane structure in the world. It is a fitting reminder that since Frei Otto designed the Munich Stadium for the German Olympics in 1972 Germany has been a major pioneer in the manufacture and use of architectural textiles. Although it is built using a conventional, doughnut-shape steel frame construction the Allianz Arena is the first building to use ETFE inflated cushions on the façade as well as the roof. They are arranged in a rhomboidal pattern, which gives the building a quilted appearance. Coloured lighting has been used to animate the membrane so that the building can respond to the events happening within it by changing its strip (red for FC Bayern Munchen and blue for TSV 1860 Munchen, the stadium's two home teams). Furthermore, the surface has been printed with a specifically designed dot matrix to give the building an opalescent finish.

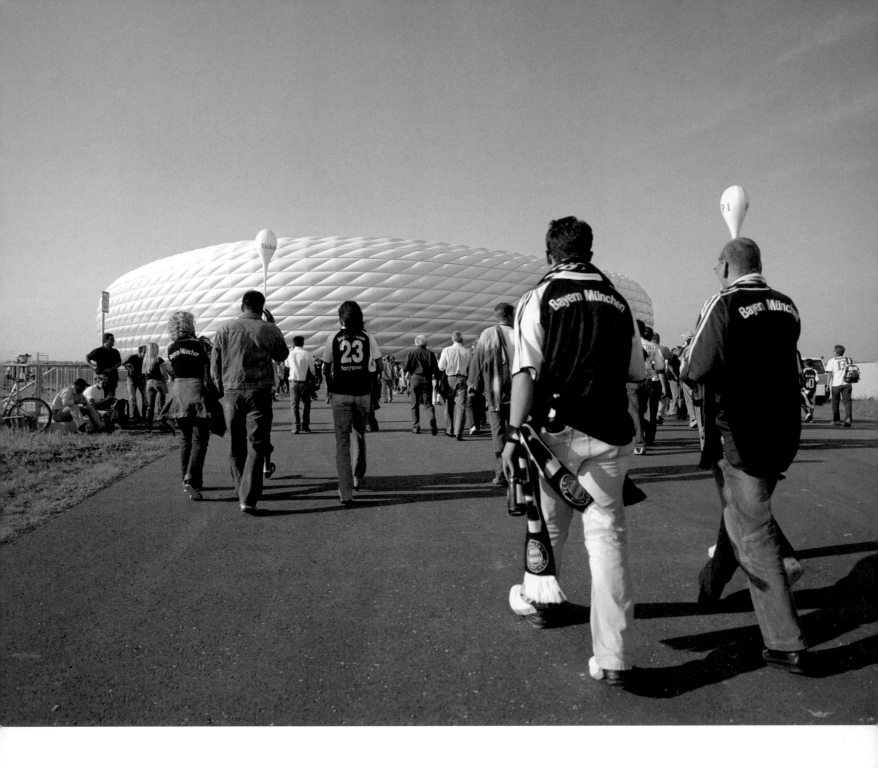

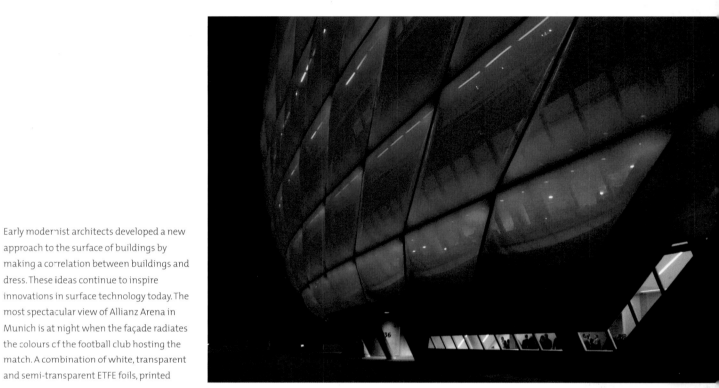

Early modernist architects developed a new approach to the surface of buildings by making a correlation between buildings and dress. These ideas continue to inspire innovations in surface technology today. The most spectacular view of Allianz Arena in Munich is at night when the façade radiates the colours of the football club hosting the match. A combination of white, transparent and semi-transparent ETFE foils, printed with a dot matrix, were prepared by the German company Covertex to give the building façade an opalescent sheen. The roof of the stadium used transparent foils which allow 95 per cent UV penetration to protect the spectators while encouraging the grass to grow.

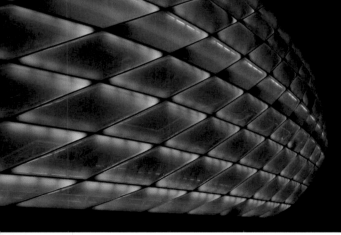

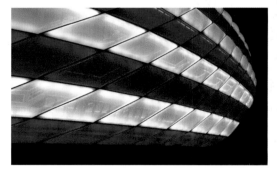

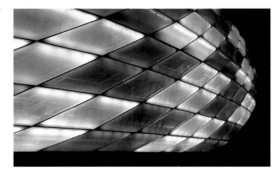

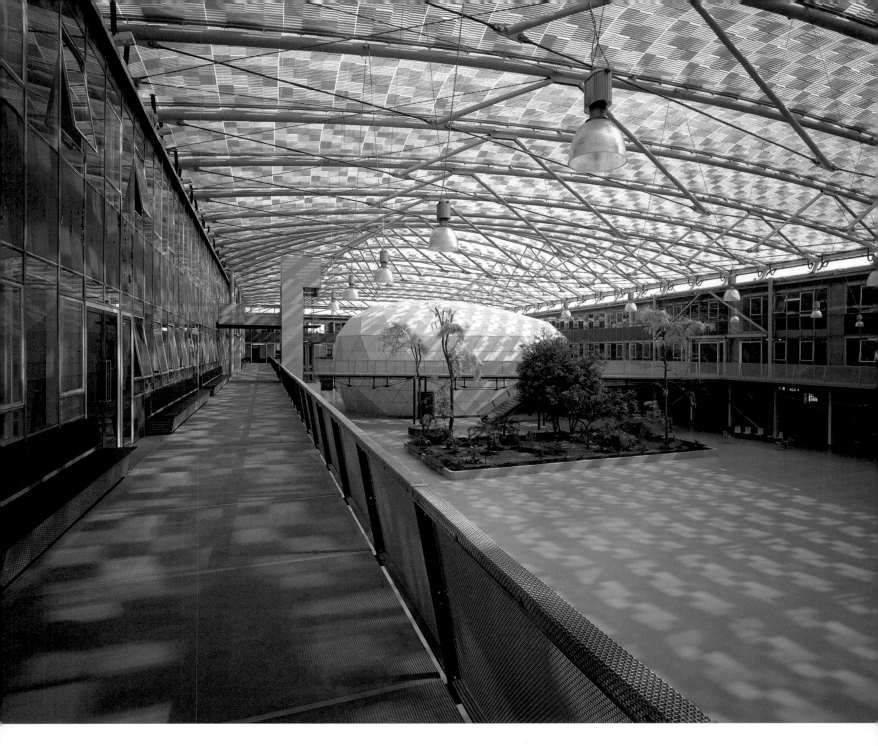

ETFE membranes have become associated with high-status projects such as sports arenas like the Beijing Water Cube, but they were used by the architectural practice de Rijke Marsh Morgan to transform the dreary schoolyard at Kingsdale School in Dulwich, London, into a multi-purpose space, equipped with a cafeteria and a theatre pod. The membrane layers are printed with coloured patterns, which appear to shift and shimmer as teachers and children move beneath them. By modifying the air pressure of the patterns screen printed on the membrane surfaces, the level of sunlight in the building can be reduced from 50 per cent to 5 per cent, converting the playground into a performance venue.

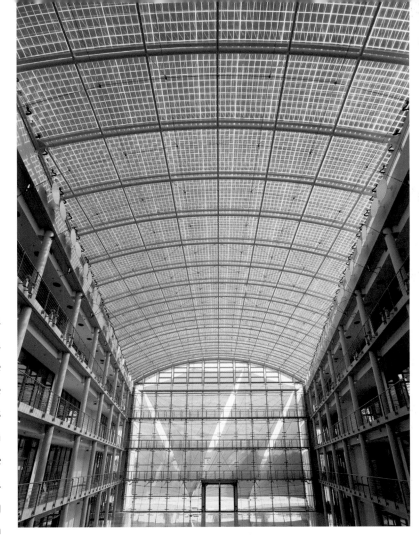

Texlon membranes printed with a chequered pattern by Vector Foiltec (UK/Germany) were commissioned in 2001 by the German architect, Ulrich Jaschek, for the atrium of the Festo Headquarters, Esslingen, Germany. They act as a sun filter.

Texlon pneumatic cushions are made up of three ETFE foils that are inflated with air to provide heat insulation. By printing positive–negative patterns on different membrane layers, the patterns can be made to overlap as the air in the cushion expands, providing shade which means that air conditioning does not need to be used.

Increasingly, architects are considering how the functions of a building can be improved through strategic surface design. For example, patterns printed on the surface of ETFE membranes can animate the interior of buildings with shadow patterns, as well as serving as a device for climatic control. By carefully positioning positive–negative patterns on both of the surfaces of an ETFE inflated cushion membrane design can be used to adjust the amount of sunlight entering a building: as the air heats up the cushions expand and the patterns start to overlap. By printing these patterns with plastic photovoltaics, light-regulating patterns may also be used as a device for gathering solar energy. Ben Morris, co-director of the Anglo-German company Vector Foiltec, which began experimenting with the use of ETFE foils as an alternative to mylar for racing yachts and pioneered the use of membranes for architecture in the mid-1980s, argues that in the future membranes will be seen as 'positive energy envelopes' – a surface that puts energy back into the world, rather than taking energy from it.

ETFE films are extremely thin (0.2 mm) and light, meaning that they are easy and cheap to transport and that savings can be made on the structure of the building. They are also extremely non-corrosive, can have a lifespan of up to thirty years and can now be recycled. Like most architectural fabrics that are waterproofed with Gore-tex, they are a bi-product of the accidental discovery of Teflon by a research chemist from DuPont Chemicals who was looking into gases for refrigeration (CFCs) in the late 1930s. Questions are now being asked by the US Environmental Protection Agency because the material used in the manufacture of Teflon, Gore-tex and other fluoropolymers (PFOA perfluoro-octanic acid) has been detected in the blood samples of members of the American population. In tests, large quantities have been shown to cause developmental problems. At the moment the traces in blood samples are small, but they are ineradicable and so there are concerns that the ongoing manufacture of these products could have an adverse effect upon human health.

New Geometries

New textile technologies are gradually changing the character and shape of buildings by allowing architects to develop their exploration of organic geometries. Architects working with tensile structures in the late 20th century were already looking for inspiration from the economy of natural forms such as spiders webs and the formation of soap bubbles. This research has now been extended through the use of computer-aided design and computer-aided manufacturing.

In the late 19th century the Irish physicist William Kelvin argued that the most economical way to divide space into cells of equal size with the least surface area between them was to make 14-sided cells (tetrakaidecahedra). Then, in 1993, Irish physicists Denis Weaire and Robert Phelan used a computer program called Surface Evolver to find an answer to the problem that improved on Kelvin's solution.

Three quarters of the cells in the Weaire-Phelan structure have 14 sides, while the rest are 12 sided; these two basic forms have been elaborated by the Australian architects, PTW, in their design for the Beijing Water Cube. Hundreds of different cushion shapes create a seemingly random, non-linear structure that is so complex it would have been impossible to build three years ago. It involves 22,000 metal tubes of different sizes.

Modernist architecture of the 20th century was largely composed of mass-produced elements. However architects working with CAD/CAM and textile composites such as carbon fibre now have the possibility of making bespoke materials that are suited to a particular project. A remarkable example of this is the 'woven office block' – a prototype that envisages how structure and surface might be fused together in the buildings of the future. The Carbon Tower prototype designed by Peter Testa and Arup, New York is a 40-storey office building of carbon fibre and composite materials. Were it to be built, it would be the lightest building of its kind in the world. The main structure is *woven* together rather than being assembled from a series of discrete parts. Forty helical bands of carbon fibre, which are 30 cm wide, 1 cm thick and hundreds of metres long, wind in both directions up the surface of the building and are clad in a double surface of translucent and transparent membranes. It is envisaged that these membranes, which would constitute the structural envelope of the building based upon a composite carbon fibre mesh, would be woven on site using new robotic and pultrusion technology. Testa and his partner Devyn Weiser have collaborated with Stephen Greenwold at MIT to design a computer tool to generate these woven meshes which are called Weaver. It allows the user to explore patterns that can be used in the building's form.

The National Swimming Centre for the 2008 Beijing Olympics, known as the Water Cube, features 100,000 sq m of ETFE foils. Designed by Australian architectural firm PTW, Ove Arup and China State Construction Engineering Corporation's Shenzhen Design Institute, the foils for the cube have been specially developed by Vector Foiltec. ETFE cushions provide good thermal insulation and they also allow 90 per cent of the sunlight to enter the building. This is used to heat the swimming pools and lowers the cost of lighting. Rain supressors have been fitted: the membrane's surface is equipped with hairs to reduce the sound of rain hitting the cushions and these anti-adhesive properties mean that rain actually cleans the building.

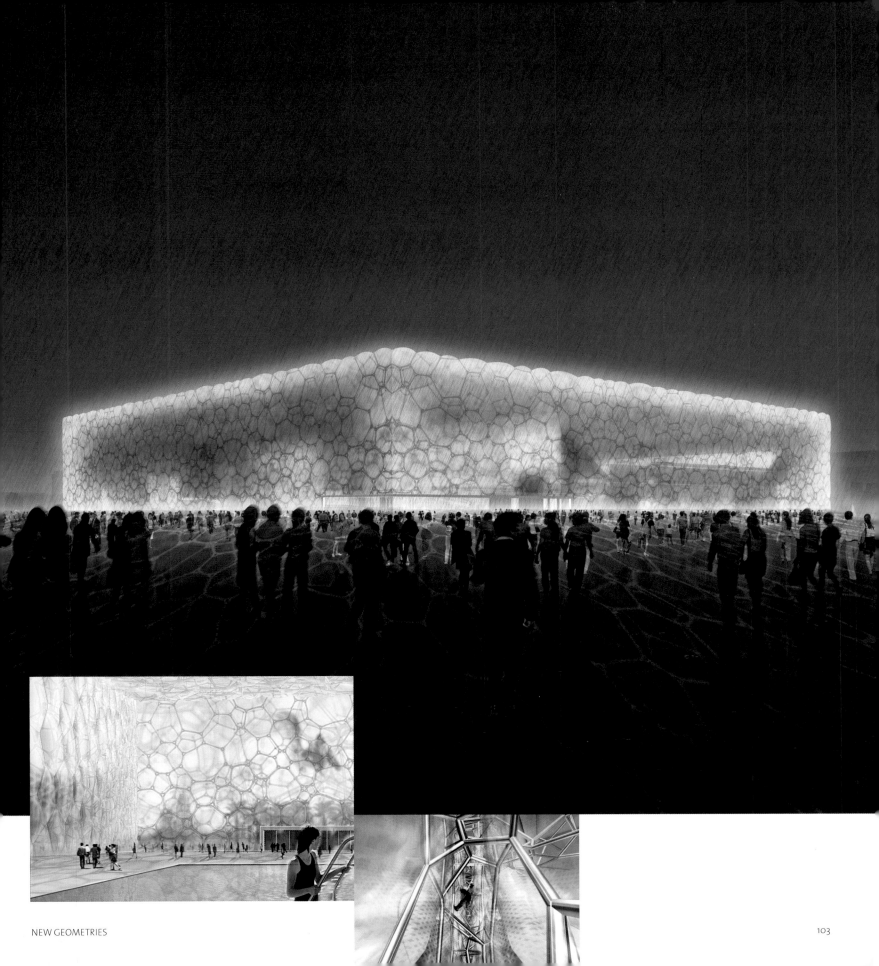

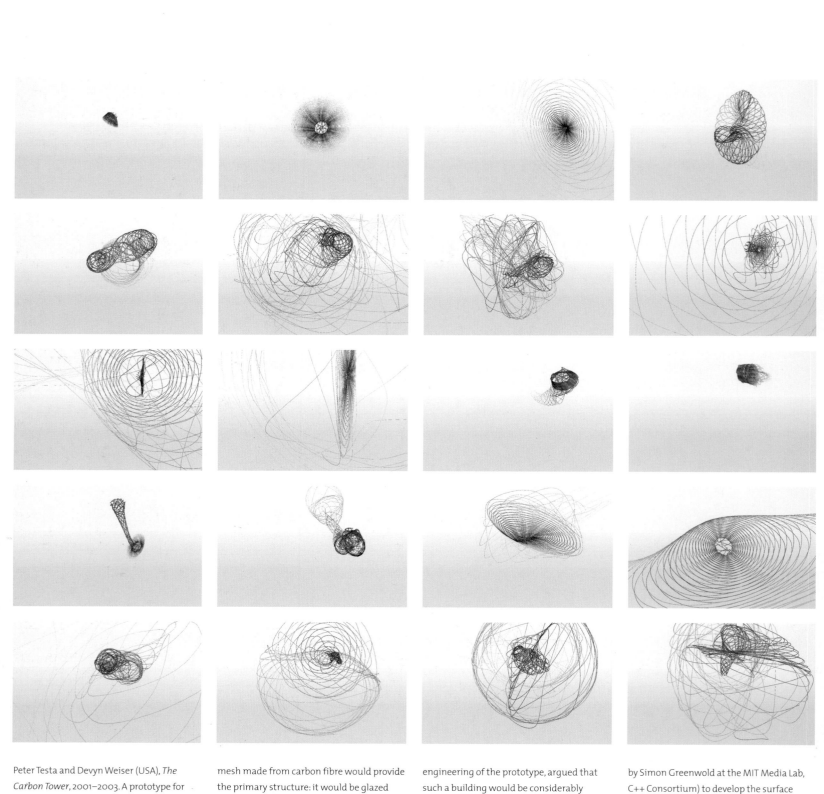

Peter Testa and Devyn Weiser (USA), *The Carbon Tower*, 2001–2003. A prototype for a circular 40-storey office building that proposes to substitute woven fibres for a conventional steel frame structure. Woven mesh made from carbon fibre would provide the primary structure: it would be glazed with membranes and composite textiles would be used for the floors. Ove Arup, New York, who assisted in the structural engineering of the prototype, argued that such a building would be considerably lighter and stronger than conventional office buildings made of concrete and steel. Testa architects used *Weaver* (developed by Simon Greenwold at the MIT Media Lab, C++ Consortium) to develop the surface structure. The programme was born out of Greenwold's research into industrial braiding and weaving techniques.

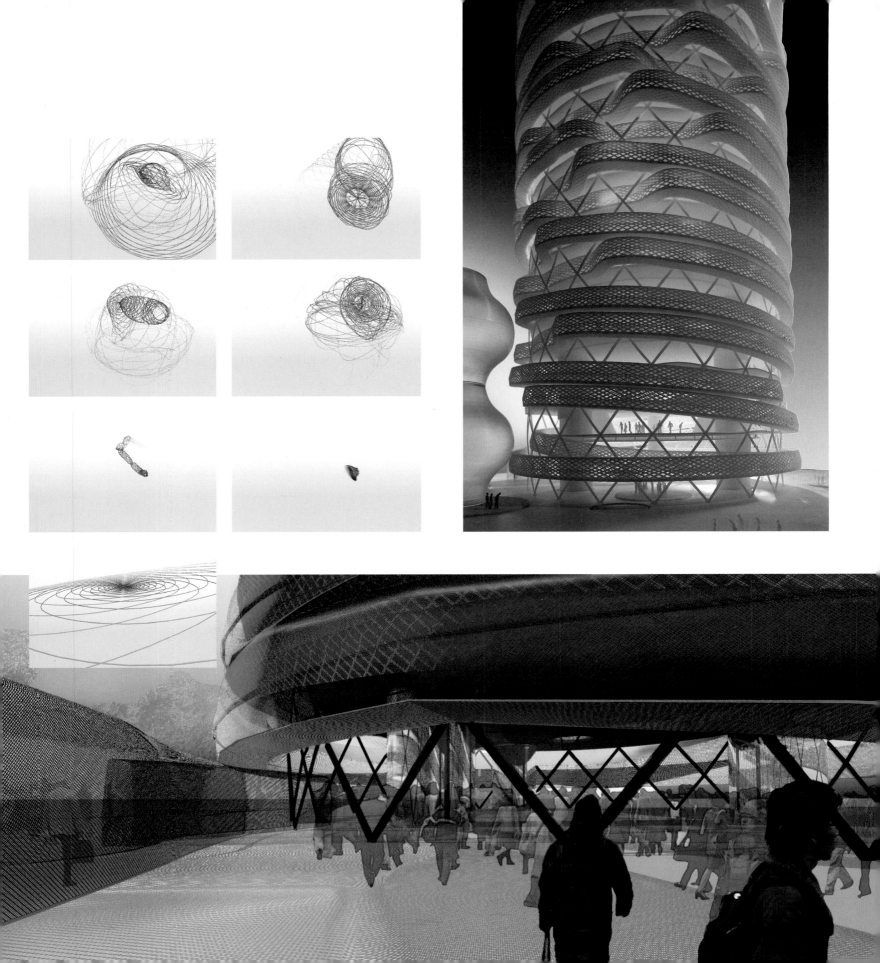

Interactive Design

Writing in 1989, George Gilder, then a leading American ideologue on the coming Information Age, proclaimed that 'the overthrow of matter' would be seen by future generations as the main achievement of the 20th century. Yet the perceived threat of cultural dematerialization seems to have prompted a widespread revival of interest in the tactile and sensory qualities of communication. In *Touch Me*, an exhibition staged at the Victoria and Albert Museum in London in 2005, the curators bemoaned the desensitization of experience: 'Many of our ordinary interactions with the world make poor use of our sense of touch. Using a computer keyboard, flicking a light switch or pushing a door provides few tactile rewards.' They exhibited a series of prototypes that they said amplified the sensory qualities of the physical and tangible world.

Maggie Orth, a former graduate in painting from the Rhode Island School of Design, was the only person with a background in making objects when computer scientists working at the media lab at MIT became fired up by ideas concerning pervasive computing in the late 1990s. 'It was a fabulous time at the lab when [computer scientists] were just beginning to question what would happen when the computer spread out into the environment. Up until that time everyone at the lab had only made things in software. I could make physical things so I became this commodity. For example, I made this rubber mould and this became the most sought after information at the Media Lab.'

Orth went on to establish International Fashion Machines to market her experimental prototypes in the field of electric textiles. She has created a series of products that explore the potential relationship between textiles lighting and colour. Initially she was interested in using textiles as an alternative format to digital display. *Dynamic Doubleweave* (2003) is a handwoven fabric over printed with thermochromic ink which changes colour when a current is applied to heat up a conductive yarn. Orth admits that she is a contrarian: 'If things were the other way round and technology was already soft I'd want to make it hard.' She enjoys working with high-tech fibres to create pieces that have a low-tech or craft look to them – a strategy that is directly analogous to Marcel Wanders' approach. Her most popular design to date is her *Pompom Light Dimmers* (2005). Made from stain-resistant, anti-microbial electronic fibre, they are touch-sensitive lights that can be adjusted by stroking and holding them.

In the IT + Textiles Project 2002–2005 conducted at the Swedish Re-form Design Studio at Göteborg, funded by the EU Disappearing Computer Initiative of the Swedish Interactive Institute, the aim was to combine smart materials with information technology. Inspired by Orth's initiative it has attempted to include conventional fabric aesthetics in these endeavours. For example, it has conducted a series of design experiments into activating pattern. *Phone Bag* by Swedish

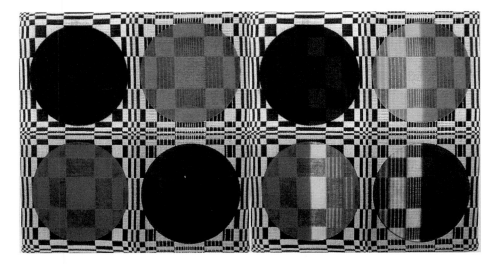

Maggie Orth (USA), *Dynamic Doubleweave*, 2003, manufactured by International Fashion Machines Inc. Cotton, rayon, conductive yarns and thermochromic ink.

Maggie Orth and Sam Bittman (USA), *Fuzzy Lightwall*, 2006, produced by International Fashion Machines Inc., and Maggie Orth, *Pompom Light Dimmers*, 2005. Orth's fuzzy light switches combine low-tech craft aesthetics with the latest conductive yarns and manufacturing techniques. Her switches are made from smart yarn that is touch-sensitive – the lights are dimmed by squeezing and stroking the pompoms. Orth became interested in interactive textiles while working at MIT's celebrated Media Lab between 1997 and 2001. These switches were manufactured by her consultancy company International Fashion Machines (IFM) which also undertakes research projects in e-textiles for private clients and the military.

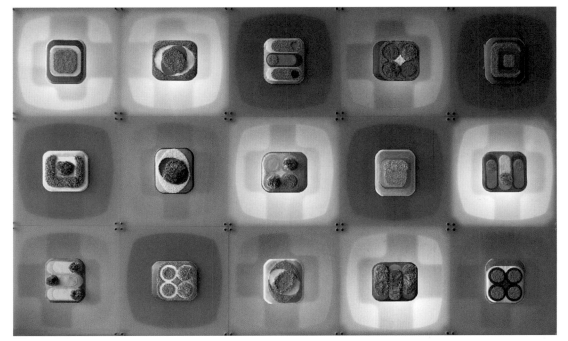

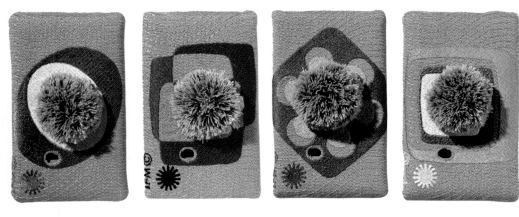

Linda Worbin (Sweden), *Phone Bag* (2005), the patterns pulse, fade and change colour when the mobile phone receives an incoming signal. The bag is made from cloth printed with thermochromic ink and woven from conductive fibres that are connected to an IT component. It forms part of the Fabrication Project, a hands-on research initiative at the Swedish school of textiles in Böras, which develops working prototypes that explore how textile aesthetics can be exploited by smart textiles.

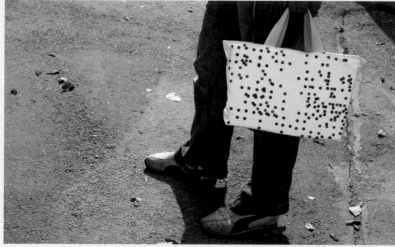

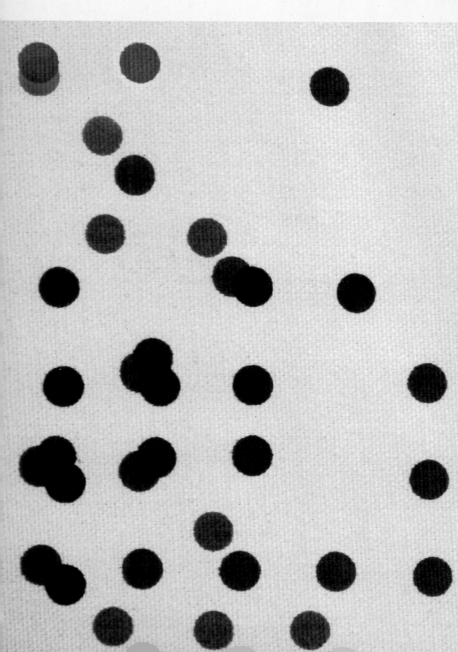

designer Linda Worbin is a prototype handbag where pulsating patterns on the bag's surface substitute the ring tones or vibration of a mobile phone. With *Tic-Tac Textiles*, a tablecloth printed with thermochromic ink becomes a canvas for studying how patterns emerge through social interaction, a couple moving coffee cups around a table. In yet another experiment, *Rather Boring Tablecloth*, printed patterns of cross-stitch emerge and disappear as heat is applied to the cloth.

The romance of sensory perception has produced a range of extraordinary concept textiles. In the *Interactive Cushion Project*, also from the Re-form studio, the patterns made from electroluminescent wire woven into homespun cushions can be activated at long range. By squeezing pillows in one location, textile patterns are activated and light up on a cushion elsewhere – an interactive device, say the designers, that overcomes the limitations of conventional telephonic communication. Another example is British designer Jenny Tillotson's *Scentsory Design* (2005), a conceptual prototype of a line of clothing integrated with computerized scent output systems.

Design experiments like these often seem destined to do little more than animate the next generation of novelty goods and toys. Yet with hindsight one can understand why textile designers inspired by research into pervasive computing (bringing the computer into the

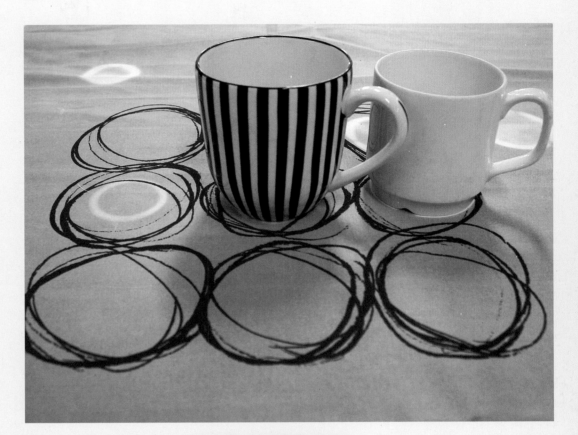

Linda Worbin (Sweden), *Tic tac Textiles*, (2004).

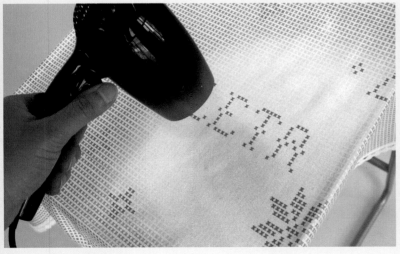

Linda Worbin and Hanna Landin (Sweden), *Rather Boring Table Cloth* (2004).

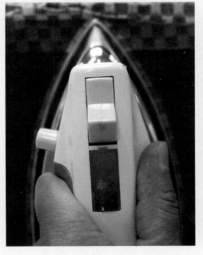

Linda Worbin (Sweden), Woven thermochromic material, 2003.

Re-form Studio, Göteborg, *Interactive Cushion* (2003). Could hugging an interactive cushion make long distance relationships more bearable? The designers of these cushions believe so. Electroluminescent wire is invisibly woven into the covers of these interactive cushions that are connected via bluetooth technology to the internet. The cushions come in pairs: the idea is that when one is touched or squeezed the other glows dynamically. The project is characteristic of the way that designers interested in pervasive computing began to investigate the affective qualities of textiles at the turn of the millennium.

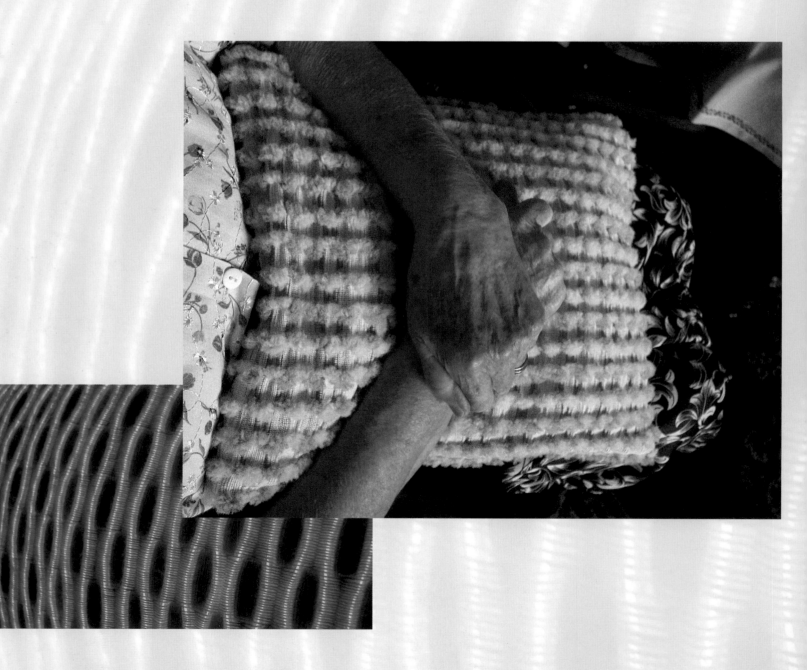

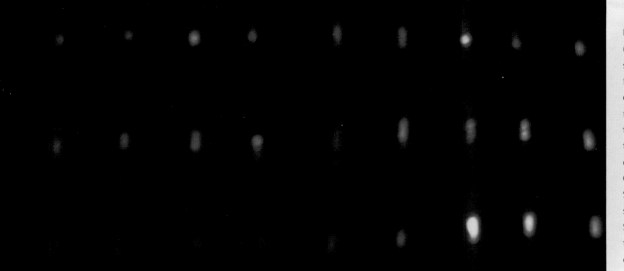

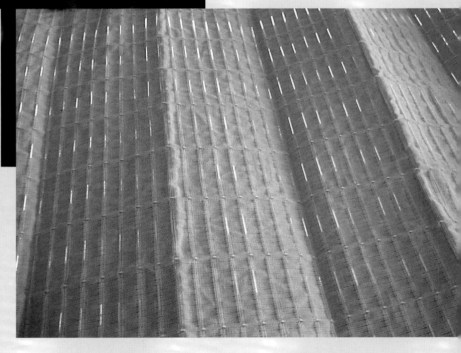

Re-form Studio, Göteborg, *Energy Curtain* (2005) is a roman blind woven with flexible solar cells and optical fibres. When the blind is drawn during the day it can harvest solar energy, which it can convert into light at night. Users can decide how much sunlight to trap, or transmit, by raising or lowering the blind. It was developed by a group of designers at the Re-form research studio in Göteborg, under the general umbrella of the Swedish Interactive Institute. The blind was shown at Static!, an exhibition mounted in Stockholm, which explored the use of design for raising awareness of energy consumption.

user's world of everyday objects) seemed to get caught up with an absurdly romantic approach to sensory or embodied experience. The concept of 'Ubiquitous computing', originally formulated by Mark Weiser in 1988 at the Xerox Park Palo Alto Research Center in California, developed at a time when the research boom into Virtual Reality (which began in the late 1980s and extended into the mid-1990s) was in full spate. Pervasive computing was a vision of the future seen from the perspective of a computer scientist who saw it as the only valid alternative for the future of the Information Society based upon virtual reality (where the user dwells largely within a computer-simulated world), which, in his view, threatened to dematerialize everyday experience.

A decade on, contemporary concerns about climate change and the limits of the world's natural resources have given us a far more earthy attitude towards textiles. They have also revived attention on how people live their lives in the real world to such an extent that Gilder's other worldly vision of a dematerialized future now seems to belong to another era. E-textiles are being adapted to make people aware of energy flows, to promote the efficient use of resources in buildings and the domestic environment. At a time when the environmental consequences of unfolding of the Industrial Revolution and mass-consumer culture to other parts of the world has begun to arouse so much concern one would have thought that modernist aesthetics would prove difficult to work with. Yet in other ways such concerns have given a utopian vision of fabric a new impetus by reinforcing the idea that adaptable fabric objects should radically change the way we live in a rich consumer culture and provide the means of social improvement in impoverished parts of the world.

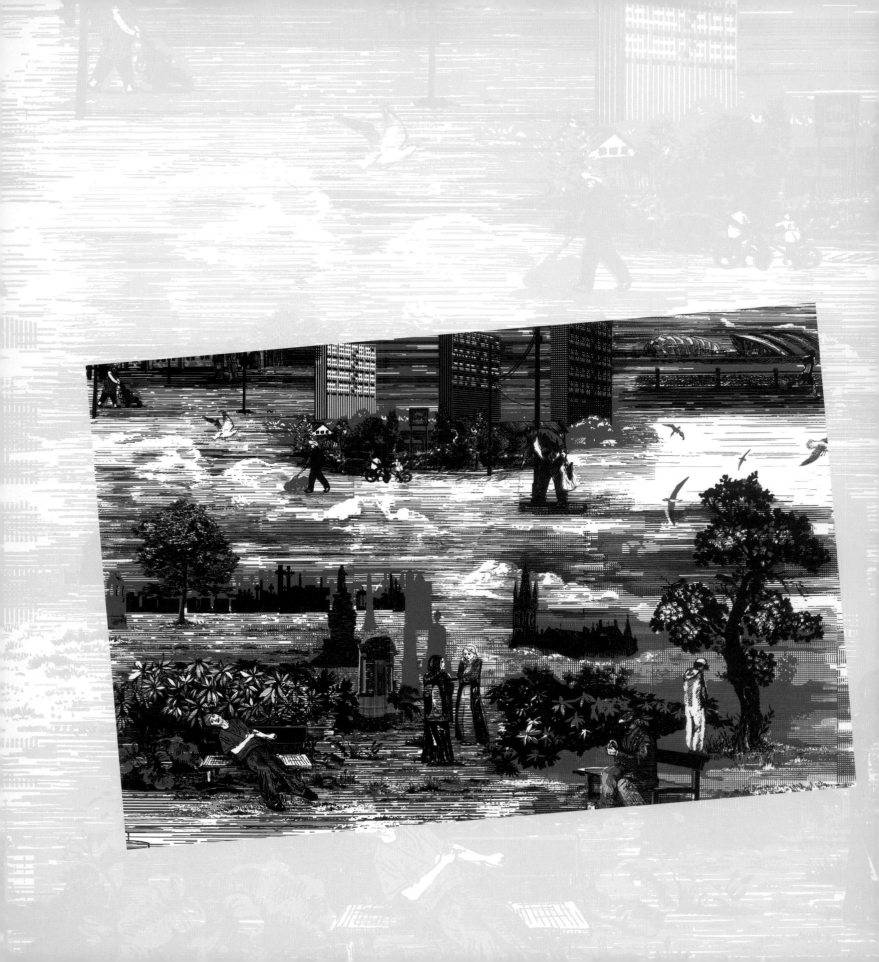

Pattern

Pattern is at once one of the most appealing and one of the most poorly understood aspects of contemporary textile design. Since the Austrian architect Adolf Loos (1870–1933) published his famous polemic *Ornament and Crime* in 1908 in which he asserted that 'the evolution of culture marches with the elimination of ornament from useful objects', the study of pattern has been marginalized within the design curricula of Euro-American contemporary design schools. Apart from Ernst Gombrich's seminal work, *The Sense of Order: A Study in the Psychology of Decorative Art* (1979), there remains little authoritative writing on the subject. Yet revivals of pattern during the 20th century present an interesting counterpoint to mainstream modernism. They indicate a range of dissatisfactions with the limitations of rational, secular modernist thought. The interest in psychedelics, which emerged from the pursuit of drug-induced mystical experiences in the 1960s and 1970s, contributed to a growth of interest in the psychology of perception and in optical effects more generally. Another example is the attraction of the East and the promise it provides of achieving alternative understandings of the nature of life's energies and ways of engaging with the psycho-physical person. Finally, archival textile patterns have presented a means of re-invoking aspects of the culture and values of the periods *preceding* 20th-century modernism. The fascination with 18th- and 19th-century archival prints re-emerged powerfully in the 1980s and remains an ongoing feature of much fabric design today.

Timorous Beasties, *Glasgow Toile* (2001), screen-printed linen.

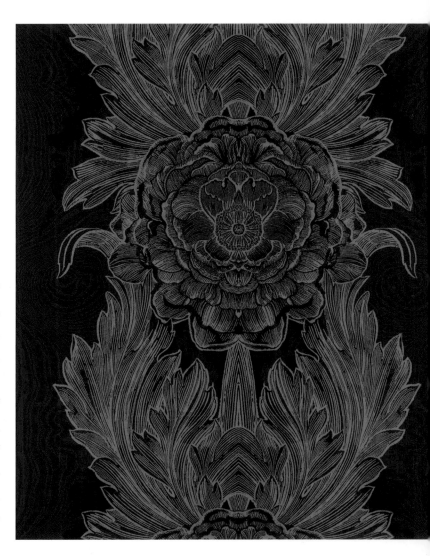

Timorous Beasties, a Glasgow-based printing studio started by Alistair McAuley and Paul Simmons in 1990, produce printed textiles that synthesize both the historicist and the countercultural tendencies discussed above. Their house style has been tellingly described as 'William Morris on acid'. In the late 1980s they achieved recognition in the design community for their surreal and provocative prints of 'beasties' derived from 19th-century scientific drawings of insects and crustaceans. They established their own print studio on the strength of this and became independent designer makers. Since then the evolution of their work has been propelled by the different cultural attitudes or cultural positions of their clients. *Glasgow Toile* (2001), the design for which they have achieved renown in the design community, grew both from their expertise in (and one senses, also their frustration at) adapting archival prints and patterns to meet the contemporary specifications of their more conventional private clients. It is a fascinating portrayal of a cultural landscape perceived by two pattern makers at the start of the 21st century.

Toiles de Jouy of the 1770s are typically associated with the depiction of Arcadian scenes of pre-revolutionary France, yet these Glaswegian designers use elements of social and political realism within them. In conversation with the Design Museum, London, McAuley

explained 'the original French 18th century *toiles*...depicted scenes... which we now see as traditional. Some scenes showed the factory at Jouy, and others rural scenes of workers relaxing, drinking and womanizing. So we did not actually change much in *Glasgow Toile*; a glass of wine became a can of super lager, a pipe became a rollie, and an old man sitting on a stool in a rural scene became a tramp on a park bench.... Some of the scenes from an area of Glasgow where we lived worked... therefore Glasgow toile seemed a perfect expression of where we were coming from.'

Timorous Beasties, *Westcoast Damask* (2004), digital and screen-printed linen. The past decade has witnessed a marked revival of interest in ornament after the minimalism of the 1990s.

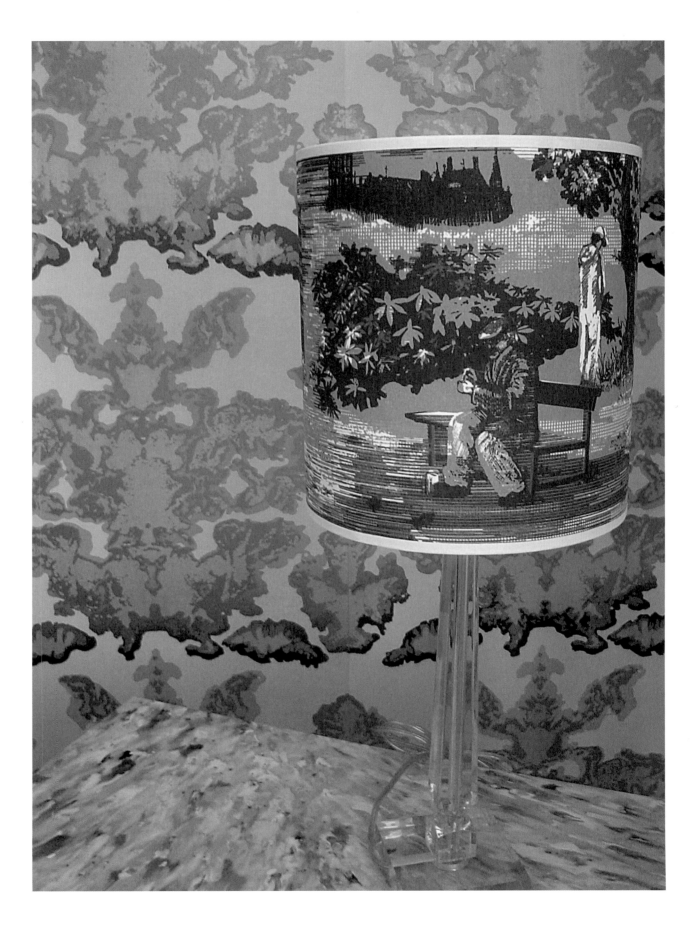

Timorous Beasties, *Toile Lamp,
Retruvious Wallpaper*, 2004.

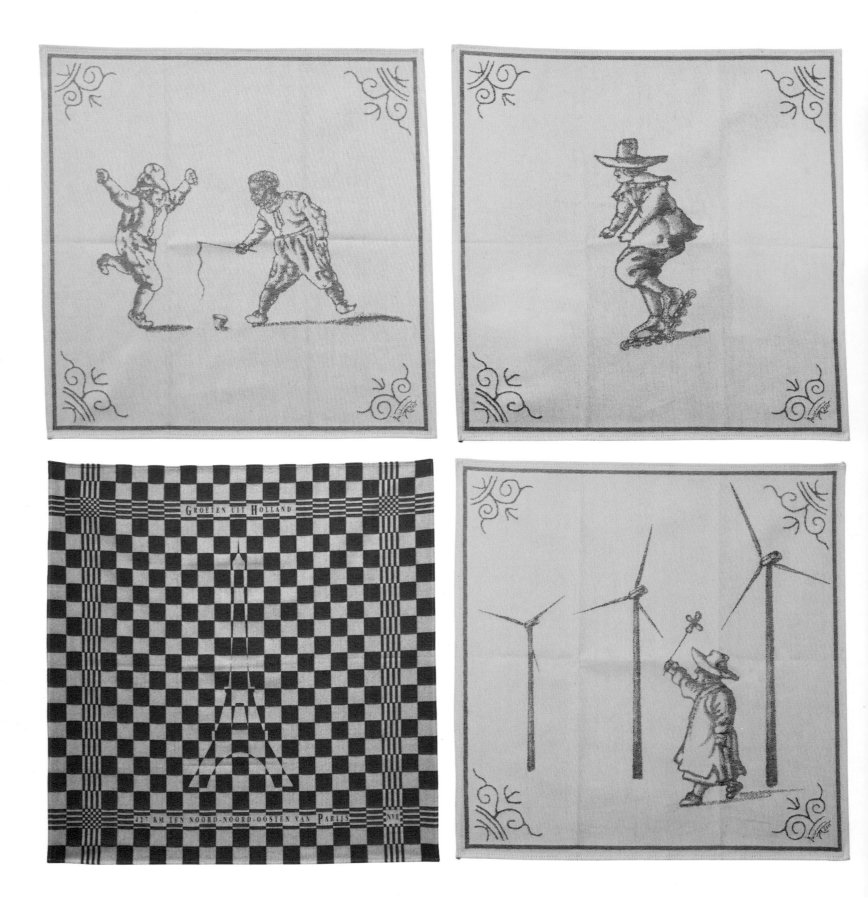

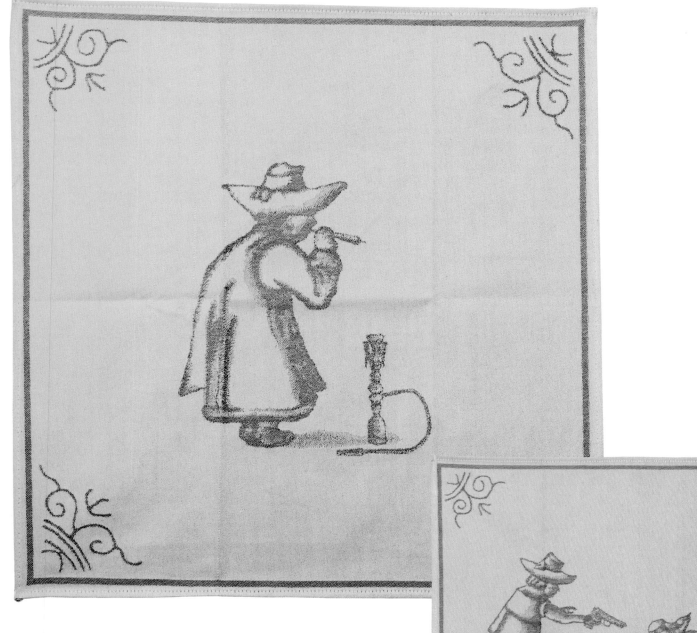

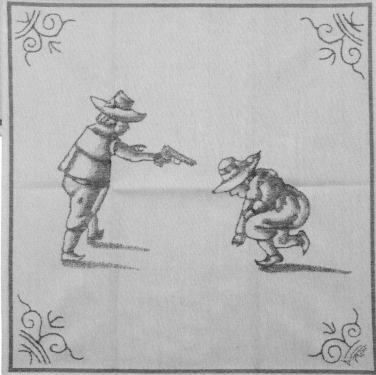

Miriam van der Lubbe (Netherlands), set
of napkin designs based on traditional Delft
tile designs, commissioned by the Dutch
Textile Museum, Tilburg, 2003.

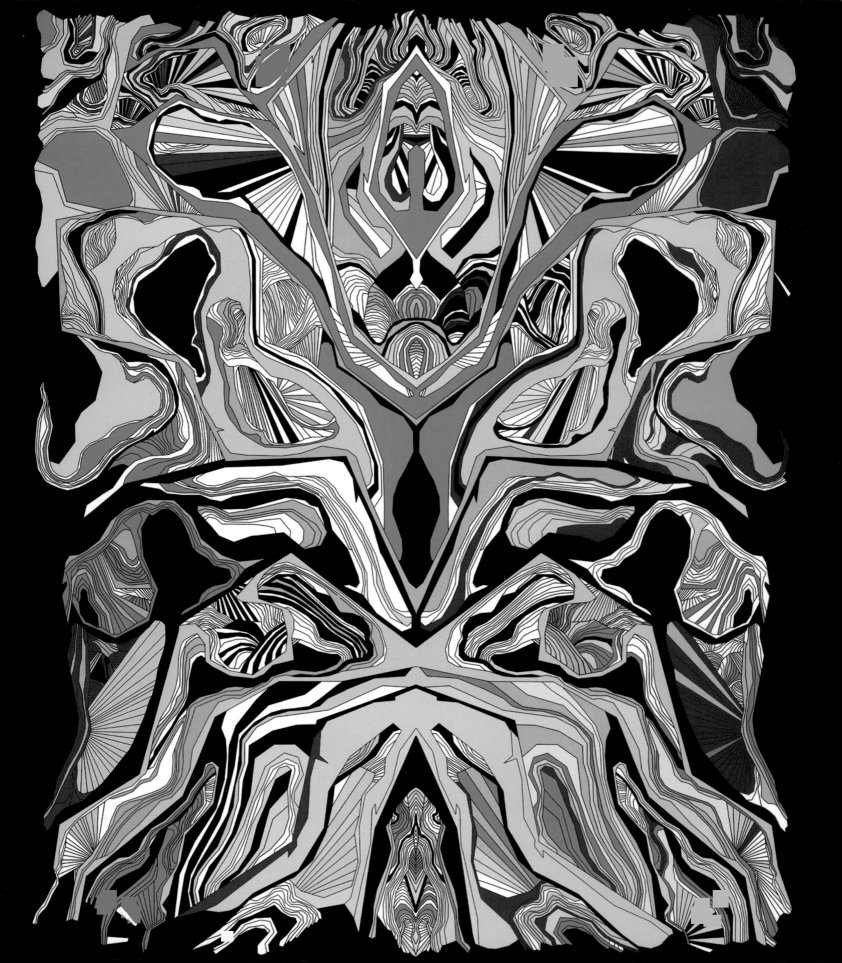

Jonathan Saunders (UK), *Wicker Pattern* (left), *Swirl Scarf* (right), *Bead Pattern* (below, right), 2005. Saunders' designs evoke a feeling of serendipity; his favoured sources of imagery have been Bauhaus-inspired graphics, ethnographic exhibits, patterns derived from Rorschach ink-blot tests and 1930s surrealist patterns. He has a three-dimensional approach to pattern: designs – often a single oversize motif – are developed for specific garments in his fashion collections. His way of working combines drawing with computer graphics and pattern making for garments: images are often projected on the wall and worked up in pencil or charcoal by hand before being reduced and digitally manipulated to fit a particular pattern. The graduated and shaded patterns are expertly screen printed by hand in his studio before being made up into frocks.

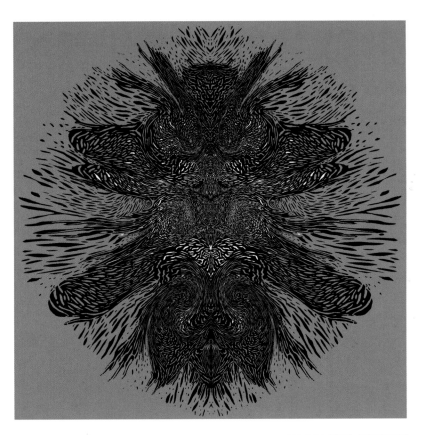

Jonathan Saunders is a more recent graduate of the department of print and textiles at the Glasgow School of Art and has established his own fashion label on the strength of his print design. In his work modernist design classics are just one of many design elements, which otherwise include ethnographic museum exhibits, scenes from contemporary pop culture and patterns from pinball machines, that are given a psychedelic twist. Saunders typically makes hand drawings of cultural artefacts that appeal to him, which he then reflects and manipulates digitally before screen printing the results on cloth by hand. As designs such as *Bauhaus Rose* (2005) show there is a kaleido-scopic aspect to the way that he adjusts the elements that he works with – it is a technique that implies that with another twist of the mill a new piece will come to the fore and a novel combination will fall into place in a different way. The patterns are large: each dress is the focal point of a single enormous motif; the pattern of tailoring and the surface pattern are considered together. This is bespoke bohemia: each print can take up to twenty screens and is specifically engineered for a single garment, one of a collection of twenty dresses.

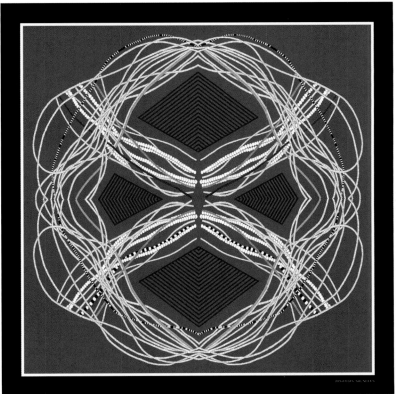

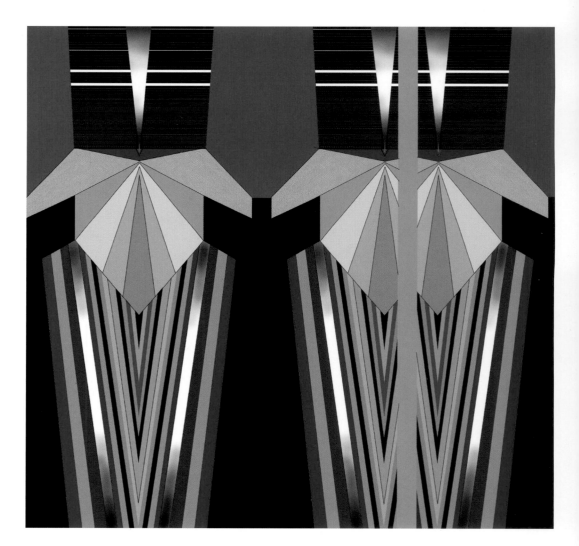

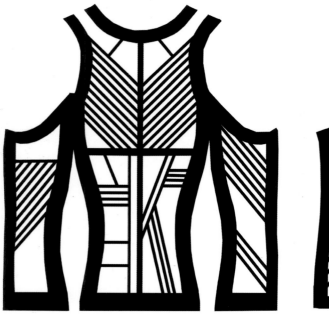

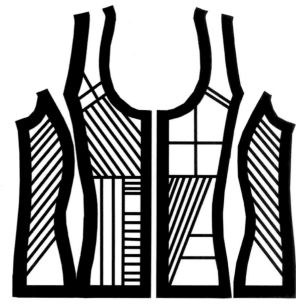

Jonathan Saunders, *Tulip Dress* (above), *Tulip Waistcoat* (left), *Two Layer Dress* (right), 2005, screen-printed designs on organza.

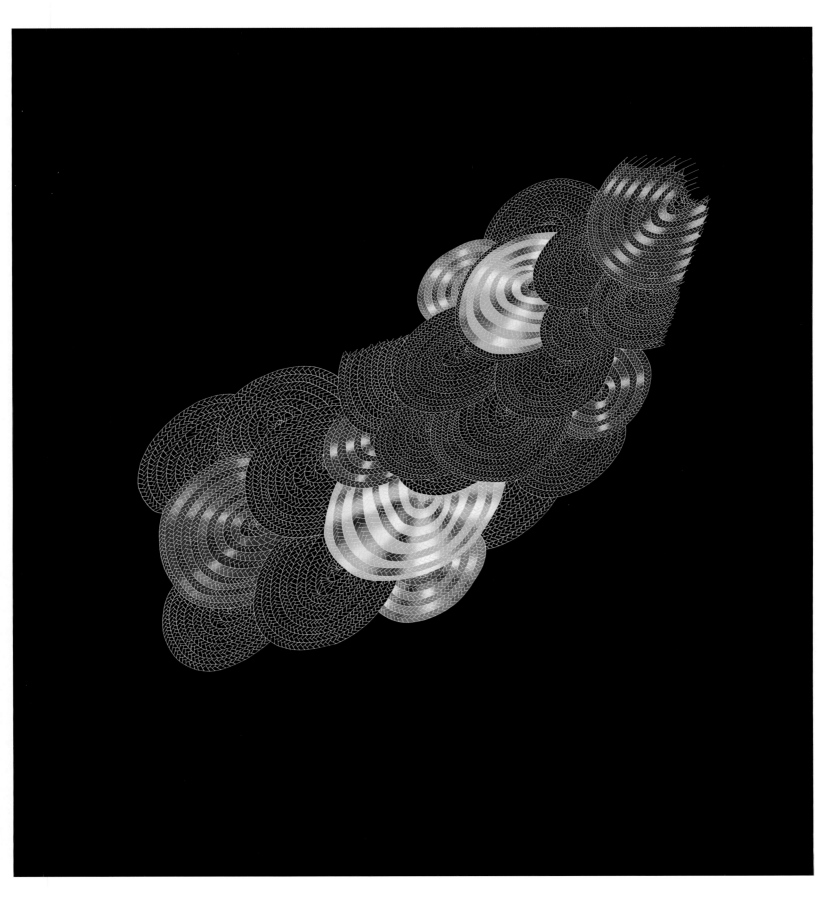

Pattern and Place

Loos' polemic was primarily targeted at Art Nouveau; the popularity of the movement was already waning by 1908 (in fact one of his primary concerns was that when an ornamental style fell out of fashion it curtailed the use of objects). It is therefore interesting to note that many of the themes of Art Nouveau – the fluid, organic forms, a certain flat, graphic quality, the adaptation of European decorative traditions by means of a foreign spatial schema (then a product of the immense excitement in Europe generated by Japanese woodblock prints) – have re-emerged as prominent concerns of contemporary 21st-century design. Design is now understood as being reinvigorated by the exchange of ideas and it is the rich, multi-cultural character of contemporary pattern and the shifting perceptions that emerge from the ongoing tumble and combination of an extensive number of different historical and contemporary cultural elements that excite our interest today.

A prime example of the multi-cultural character of contemporary pattern can be found in the work of the London-based design studio founded by Mark Eley and Wakako Kishimoto. Eley Kishimoto produce patterns that are so powerfully formed they create a perceptual shadow in the mind, leaving one re-sensitized to the patterns that surround one. Their patterns are bold and clean, the shapes simplified and the scale enlarged, and they are rendered with the minimum number of colours – for practical reasons, they insist. It was this economy that helped them to establish a fashion label from their hand-printed fabrics. They favour designs that seem familiar because they draw upon everyday things: the graphic prints found on 1970s drip-dry shirts; a tea towel that identifies different nautical knots; flock wallpaper; household cleaners.

Many Eley Kishimoto patterns evoke styles of ornament such as Art Nouveau, or Op Art, which point to the *history* of the exchange of ideas between the East and the West. The resultant syntheses leap beyond national parochialism by making one see familiar, regional patterns in a new, more international way. In *Landscape* (2003) the rolling English countryside achieves a new kind of fluidity that is at once familiar and foreign. These designs are both formal and cultural in the widest sense: references to history or high culture are offset by Wakako's self-professed love of cartoon graphics and kitsch, but these elements are brought together and harmonized with immense economy. In their signature design, *Flash* (2001), the easy domestic associations of the pattern (taken from the graphics of the floor cleaner of the same name) are packed with an optical charge that seems to engage directly with the way that the eye makes sense of visual appearance.

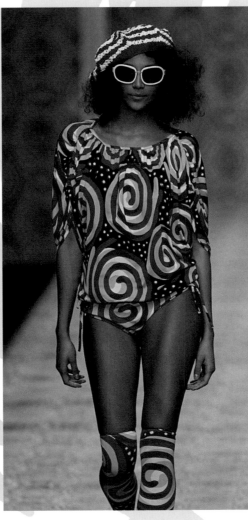

Eley Kishimoto (UK), *Big Spin*, Spring/
Summer 2005.

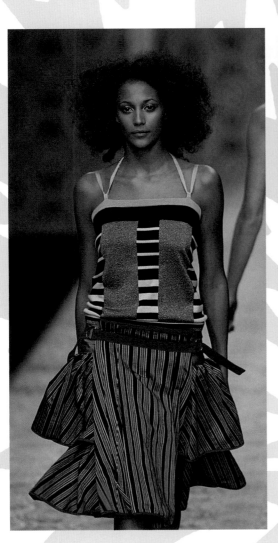

Eley Kishimoto (UK), stripy lurex knit tank
and woven side ruffle skirt, Spring/Summer
2005.

Eley Kishimoto (UK), *Domino Butterfly*, Summer 2004.

Eley Kishimoto (UK), *Ropey*, Summer 2002.

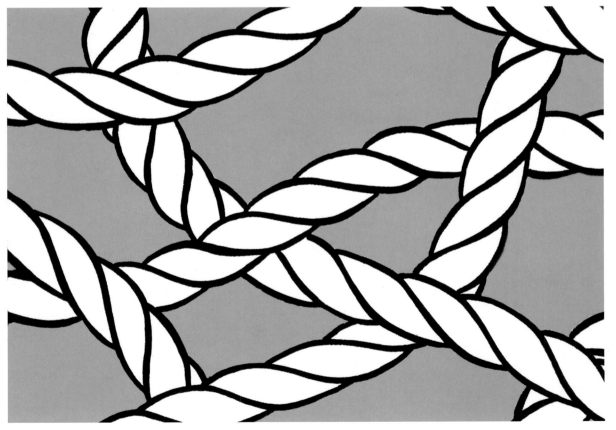

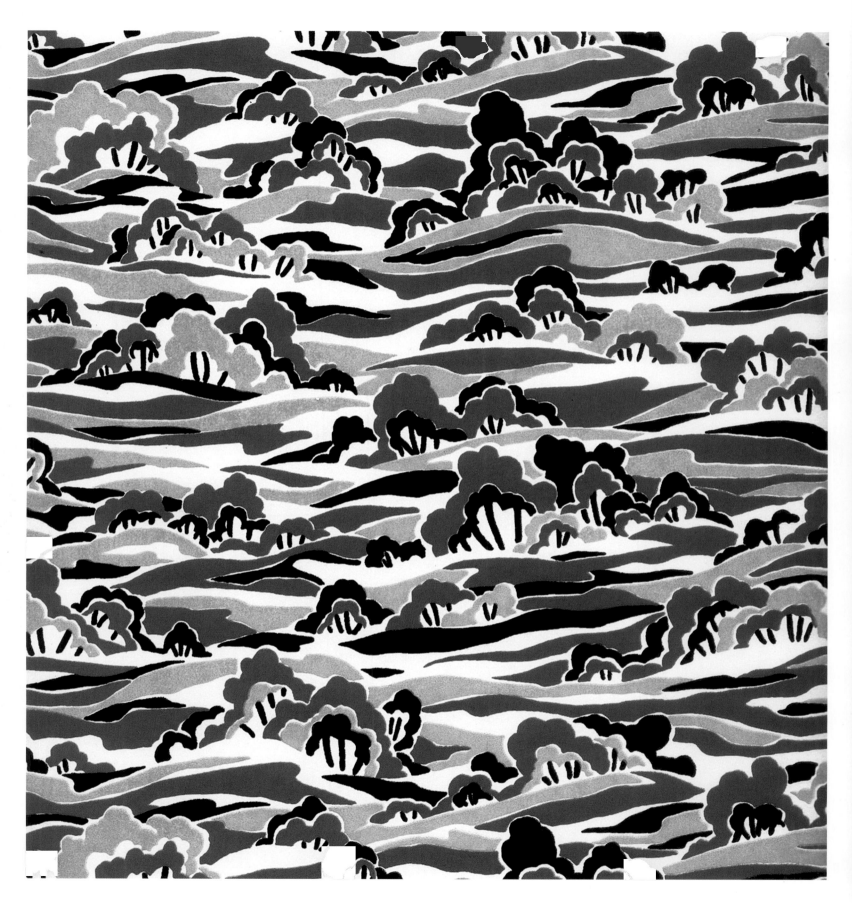

Eley Kishimoto (UK), *Blue Landscc pe*, Winter
2001/2002.

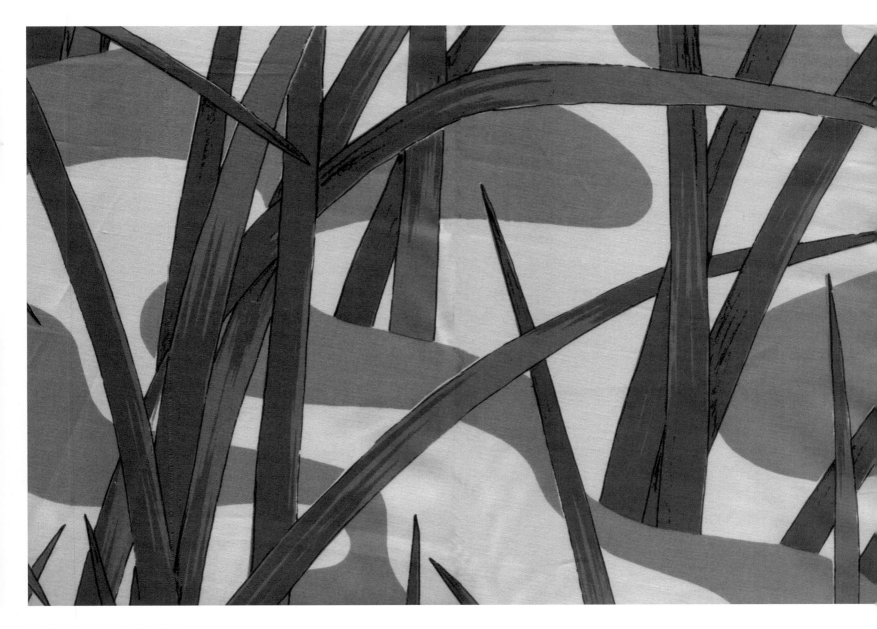

Eley Kishimoto (UK), *Marshland*, Wi⁊ter
2004/2005.

In Paris, international influence, like street style, has tended to be refracted through the perception of European designers of prêt à porter and couture, who perceive the world at one, or perhaps two removes through the inspiration of illustrated books and exhibitions, and other media. But in the late 1980s Parisian clothing found a champion in the Malian designer Lamine Badian Kouyaté (born 1962). Since he launched his label in 1989, his cosmopolitan clothes, cut and recombined from second-hand clothing and other materials (Chitenge cloth, tie dye, T-shirts, Army Coats, knitwear, fun fur, lace) sourced in the streets and flea markets of Paris, have focused the attention of the international fashion press on the cosmopolitan character of Paris's streets. His Summer 2006 collection, *100% Recycled*, consists of second-hand Hawaiian shirts or African wax prints that are overprinted with bold graphics in gold leaf.

Kouyaté was born in Bamako, but his mother is from Senegal. The name of his label, Xuly Bët (which means 'keep your eyes open' in Wolof), conveys the idea that the future is on your doorstep – it is about a new approach to the here and now; it conveys his ambition to make people open to their immediate surroundings. The directness of his approach – the fact that he works with the fabric to hand – makes it tempting to draw a parallel with the famous Malian women's tradition of Bogolan,

where locally grown cotton is coloured by being immersed in local materials such as tree sap and mud. But the analogy seems inappropriate, not least because Kouyaté's clothing tends to incorporate synthetic fabrics that have been tie-dyed in Senegal. A stronger analogy might be found between Xuly Bët and the cosmopolitanism of Bamako itself, where French clothing, combined with fabrics traded from other parts of West Africa, Morocco and Algeria, created the distinctive Bamako approach to style during the 1960s and 1970s, brilliantly conveyed by local photographers such as Seydou Keïta and Malick Sidibé.

Cut and mix is one approach to combining fabrics, but pattern itself is attractive: it allows pattern makers to connect disparately sourced material by discovering similarities of form between different motifs. It is the appealing, 'cognitively sticky' character of pattern that fascinated the anthropologist Alfred Gell, who suggested that this quality is conveyed by the adjective 'tacky', the term pejoratively used to dismiss hippy patterns in the late 1970s.

A slightly tacky approach to pattern is an important aspect of the work of New Delhi-based fashion designer Manish Arora whose richly patterned and embroidered fusion fashions for his Winter 2006/2007 collection were based upon the idea of a particular flight of fancy –

Xuly Bët (Lamine Badian Kouyaté), Mali/France, from the *100% Recycled collection*, 2006. Xuly Bët means 'keep your eyes open' or 'be alert' in Wolof, a language spoken in Senegal. Looking at Xuly Bët's work is an invitation to see, almost with his eyes, the relationship between particular fabrics and the quarters in the north of Paris where the immigrant communities from North Africa live and work. Nearly all the fabrics that Xuly Bët works with – African wax prints, fun fur and lace – are initially sourced from the flea markets close to his workshop before being patched, over printed and made into new garments. Here, a second-hand Hawaiian shirt, sourced in the Marché de Clignancourt, is screen printed with gold with a positive–negative pattern that allows the words 'Xuly Bët Funkin' Club' to emerge from the cloth.

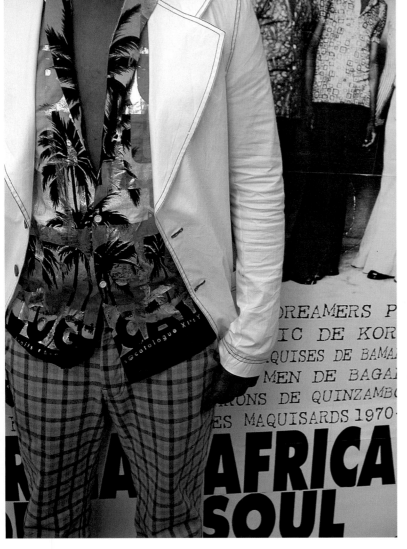

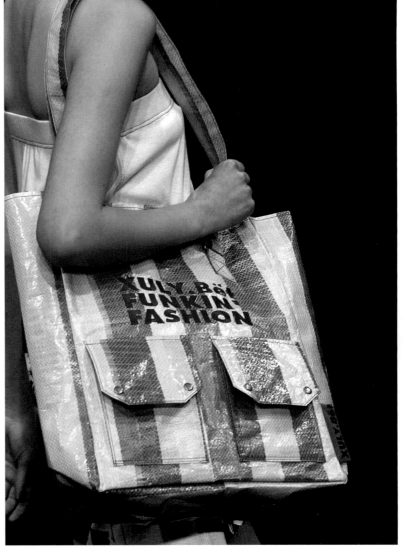

'A trip to visit Father Christmas in Lapland via Bombay, London, Japan and Russia'. Arora likes the pink, green, orange, turquoise and kitsch and confusion of the Bombay streets, where he grew up. 'Every country has aspects of its culture that it prefers not to see because people don't consider them good taste, but often they are the things that other nations appreciate about you. I love India's kitsch side and it's a big part of my work', says Arora, who held his first fashion show in 1997 and has emerged as India's best-selling prêt-à-porter designer, much favoured in the Bollywood scene. 'Now it seems that many other Indians are ready to embrace it too.'

Arora is widely regarded as the pioneer of contemporary Indian fashion design. Until a decade ago, this was largely restricted to toned-down, conservative, Mughal-inspired couture and traditional wedding clothes for the domestic market and the cheap, cheese-cloth dresses exported for sale in ethnic shops and street markets elsewhere. Arora's designs are at once international in scope (not simply in terms of reference but market, he exhibits at London fashion week and his label is sold internationally), while being a symptom of the new urban consumer culture that is developing on the streets of Mumbai and New Delhi. His internationalism is not new: European designers have

Xuly Bët (Lamine Badian Kouyaté), *PVC Barbès*, customised PVC travel sac from the *100% Recycled collection*, 2006. Chequered PVC travel sacs are a familiar a sight on the streets around Barbès-Rochechouart, the old Arab quarter of Paris where settlers from North and West Africa congregate.

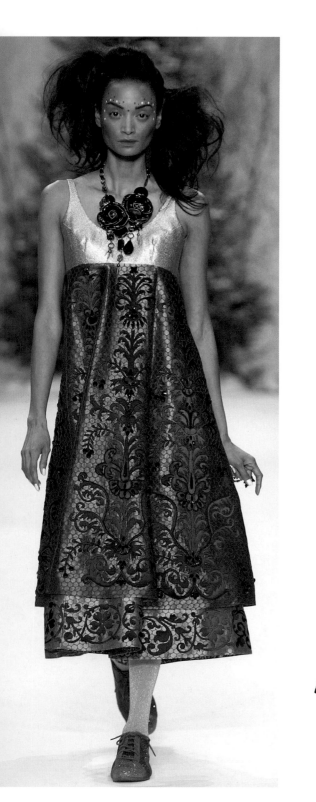
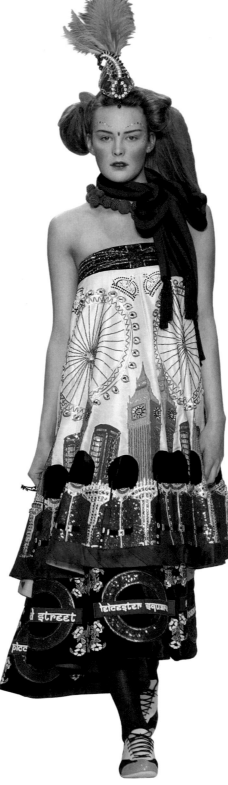
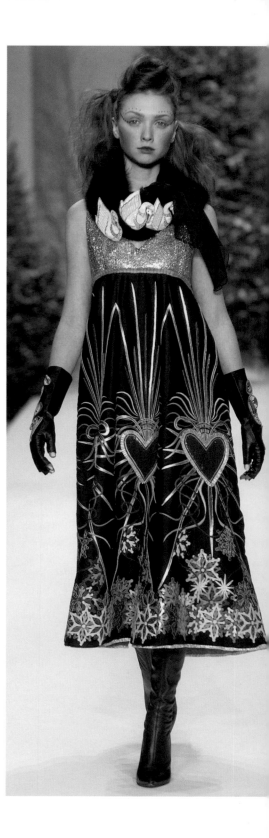

Manish Arora (India), *Dreaming* (left), *London* (centre), *Love* (right), from the Winter 2006/2007 collection. Arora has shown three collections at London Fashion Week. He was the first Indian fashion designer to launch an international luxury brand. Based in New Delhi, his clothing is densely ornamented and hand embroidered.

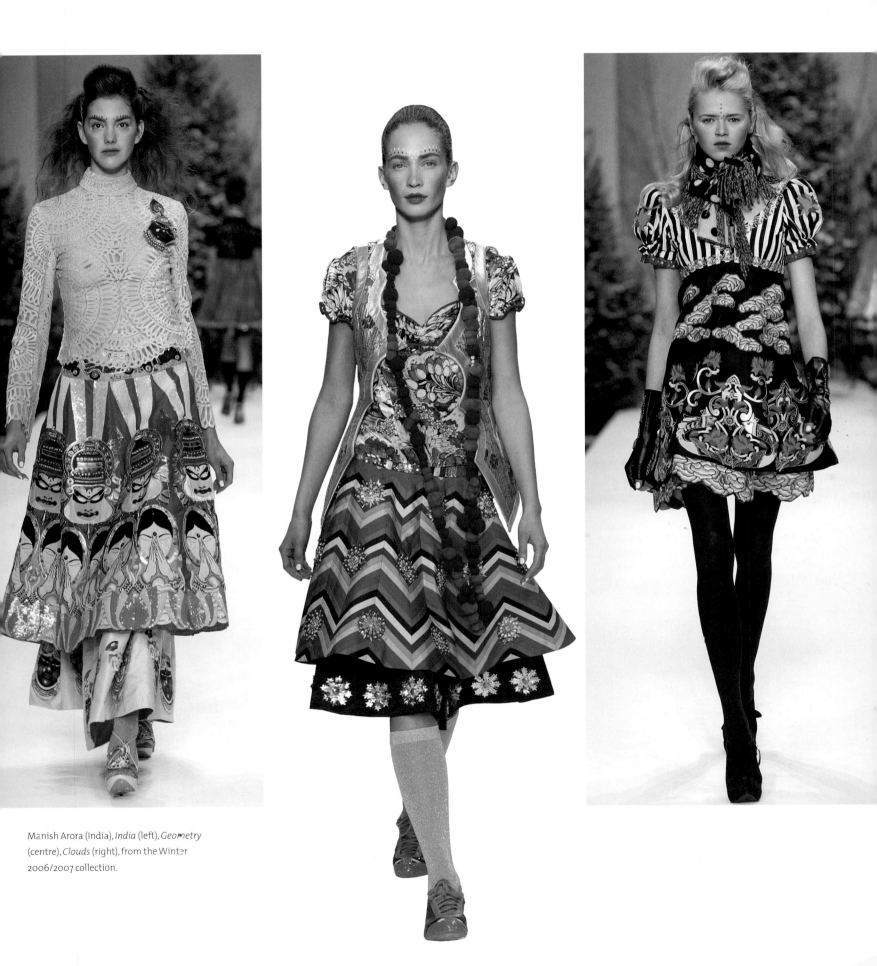

Manish Arora (India), *India* (left), *Geometry* (centre), *Clouds* (right), from the Winter 2006/2007 collection.

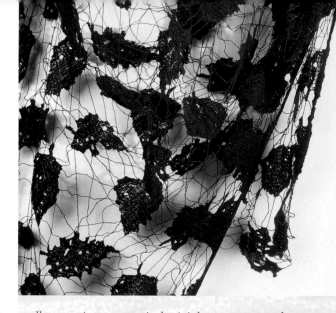

often been inspired by Indian styles, he remarks disingenuously, since it is designers like him who may transform the world of textiles and fashion in the 21st century by tipping the topography of the market towards the East.

In contrast to these new designers who draw upon the cosmopolitan character of textile traditions and urban clothing in cities across the world, Japan, the first East Asian country to become an independent fashion capital, is celebrated for having a distinctively different approach, where many of its most celebrated textile designers combine distinctive local textile traditions, developed during Japan's long period of isolation, with contemporary textile technologies.

Reiko Sudo formed NUNO in 1984 with the renowned Japanese textile designer Junichi Arai. Sudo's work for the NUNO Corporation is securely located *within* the traditions of Japanese craft textiles which she stretches to the limit by using contemporary technology. This small corporation of designers and technicians has produced 14,000 fabrics which fuse traditional craft techniques with innovative finishing processes. NUNO take their inspiration from Japanese craft traditions and materials, such as Okinawa banana fibre, or the silk-weaving traditions of Amami-Oshima island, or conventions of origami folding, as

well as contemporary industrial processes such as spray painting for the automobile industry. The emphasis is upon material and process and the way fabrics feel as opposed to cultural representation. As the names of different fabrics show: *Brickyards, Bubble Pack, Slipstream, Graffiti, Shutter* (inspired by the roll-down shutters used to protect the plate glass windows of shops at night), *Fan* or *Kareha* (lit. 'leaf skeleton' in Japanese), patterns are typically inspired by features of the urban cityscape that are selected more for their formal or textural character than as representations of aspects of contemporary Japanese culture. During the course of the 1990s they developed patterns and surface texture through pushing existing techniques of fabric manufacture to its limits by systematically breaking the rules: yarns were overspun; jacquards were developed to the limit of complexity into dense, multilayered cloths using CAD/CAM; yarns of incompatible shrinkage were deliberately combined and heat treated to produce strange crinkled effects. In the 1990s NUNO emerged at the forefront of the revival of interest in devoré and the chemical treatment of cloth. Fabrics were eroded with chemical etching, polyester was even put in the microwave; however, more recently they have renewed their interest in sustainable design.

Reiko Sudo, engineer, and Yoko Ando, surface designer (Japan), *Kareha (Leaf Skeletons)*, 1998. Made up of 65% acrylic, 25% wool and 10% rayon. Patterns are machine embroidered onto a thin, soluble substrate, which is then dissolved, leaving a lace-like openwork fabric. Due to environmental concerns, NUNO Corporation, the manufacturer, now use water-soluble materials such as vinylon to achieve similar effects.

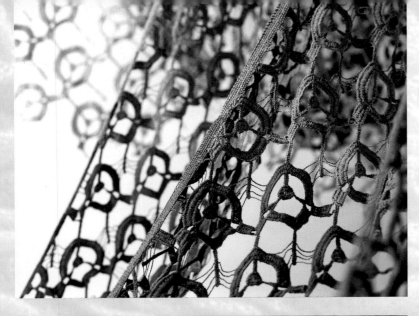

Reiko Sudo (Japan), *Electric Fan*, 2000, 70% cotton, 30% rayon. A pattern of an old-fashioned electric fan is embroidered onto a base fabric, which is then dissolved using a strong alkali solution, leaving only embroidered motifs interconnected by a fine network of threads. Junichi Arai and Reiko Sudo established the NUNO textile design studio in 1984. As the firm's name implies (nuno means cloth in Japanese), the approach is artisanal: the fabrics are not mass produced, but are serially made and are characterized by the inventive use of synthetics and industrial processing techniques.

Reiko Sudo and Tomoko Miura (Japan), *Tanabata*, 2004, from the *Origami Pleats Series* manufactured by the NUNO Corporation. Sudo made *Tanabata* by sandwiching a length of polyester organza between two differently coloured heat-transfer printing papers. It is carefully folded using an origami technique and then heat set and heat cut in a vacuum-transfer machine. The heat subliminates the dye onto the cloth, permanently impresses the polyester with the folded pattern and is used to cut the fabric, making it mobile. When it is worn as a scarf, the folds shift and change as if with their own dynamic.

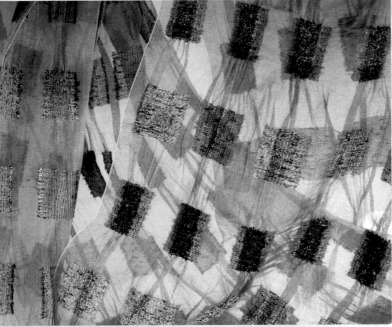

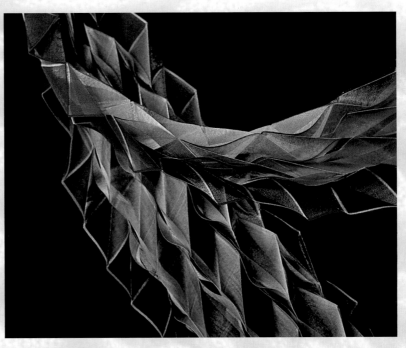

Reiko Sudo (Japan), *Re-Text*, 2003. Made of waste threads left over from the production of Oshima Tsumugi, a silk, ikat-dyed fabric that is used to make bespoke kimonos on Amami Oshima island. To prepare this fabric, threads are bound with cotton before being dyed with plant materials, indigo and mud. Once they are mounted on the loom, the warp threads need to be positioned carefully in order to achieve delicate figurative kimono designs, a process that yields a good deal of waste threads. These threads are collected, re-spun and used at the NUNO Corporation to make new yarns which are then jacquard woven into cloth.

Karina Nielsen (Denmark), *Leno Weave*, 2004.

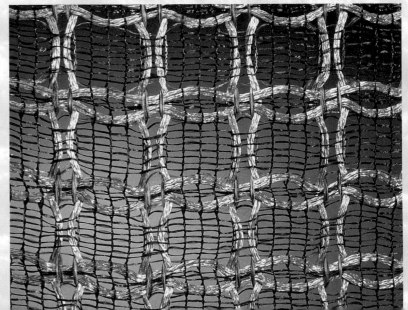

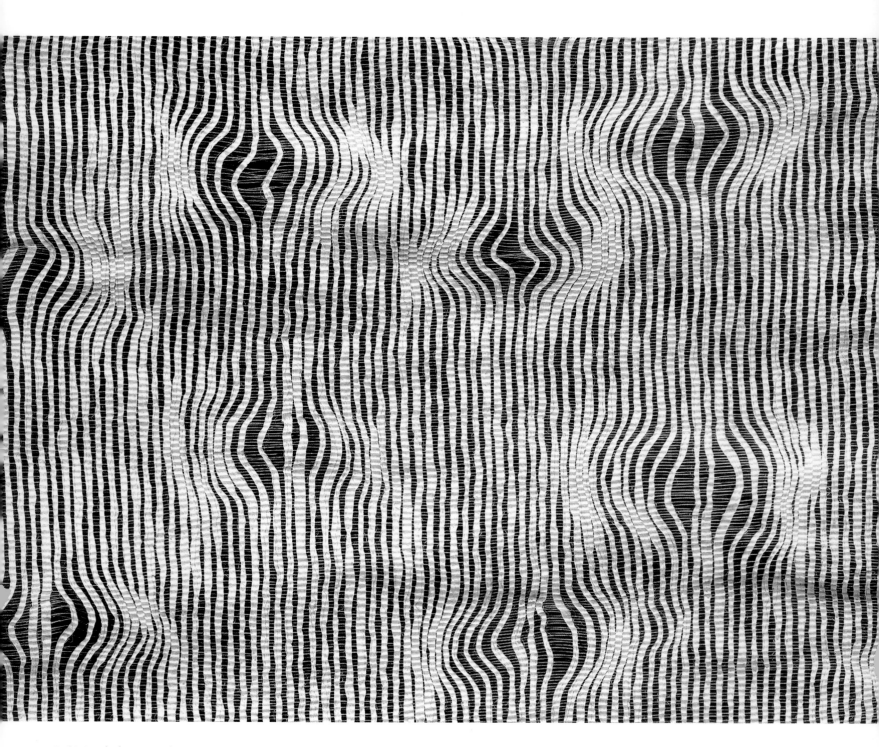

Sophie Roet (UK), *Paper Textile*, 2004. Designed to be suspended in front of a window and looks like a paper cobweb when it is seen at night. It was woven on a rapia loom in West Yorkshire in England, using a transparent polyester warp. The paper wefts are manipulated by hand to create the gentle movement of the stripes. Roet was born in Australia and is a contemporary textile designer who has an interest in both traditional craftsmanship as well as contemporary industrial textiles and experimental materials such as paper and metal. For her new venture R and B enterprises, launched in 2005, she has collaborated with craft specialists based in Kolkata (formerly Calcutta) in India to create a collection of woven, printed and embroidered fabrics.

Sophie Roet (UK), *Scattered Flowers*, 2005. A metal coil solma is fastened onto the cloth in an abstract organic form.

Sophie Roet (UK), *Metal Flowers*, 2005. Hand-embroidered onto silk crepe fabric using metal thread in Kolkata, India. The embroidery is then beaten into the fabric so that it becomes embedded.

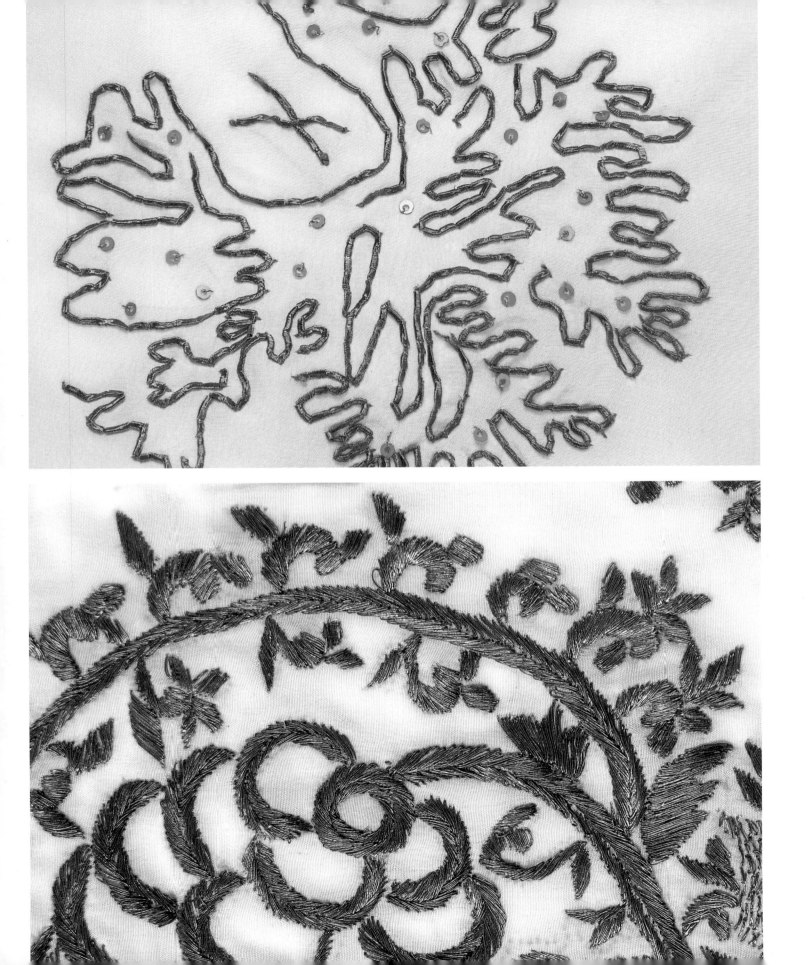

Pattern, Perception and Form

The cultural and political bias of much recent work with highly pattern-ed textiles makes it almost shocking to find a non-Western designer whose textiles are comparatively abstract and concerned with issues of texture and form. Joel Adrianomearisoa, who entered the Fashion Academy of Antananarivo in Madagascar at the age of 12, before moving to Paris to study architecture in 1998, experiments with wood, metal, stone and plastics – materials usually associated with sculpture – to create object-garments mostly rendered in a palette of blacks. There is a strong cultural component to his architectural approach to cloth.

Experiments with formal abstraction, as shown in French and Italian 18th- and 19th-century textile archives, were a prominent feature of textile design *prior* to the emergence of modern movements of formalist art such as minimalism. What distinguished these experi-ments was, of course, the context of their production and their scale: most of these designs could still be labelled decorative because they were small. Issues of scale also play an important part in the spatial perception of pattern in domestic interiors. Patterned textiles have often had some difficulty fitting into the classic modern interior. This is as much a problem of form, to do with figure-ground relations as anything else: white walls delineate the contours of pieces of furniture so forcefully that they begin to act as motifs, meaning that the primary

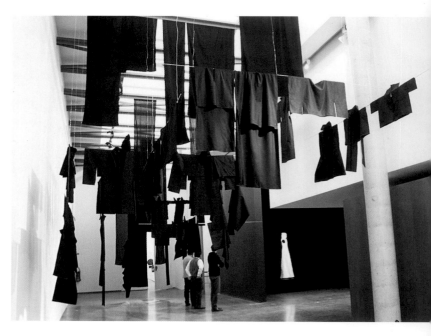

spatial dynamic occurs at the scale of the room. By contrast, coloured or patterned walls mean that the contours recede and the primary dynamic is more muted and accented by the interaction of many smaller patterns. Such issues have contributed to a contemporary phenomenon described by Peter York as 'pillow proliferation', where designers such as Anne Kyyrö Quinn use enlarged motifs, in her case, on her cushion covers, to make their designs work in minimalist interiors.

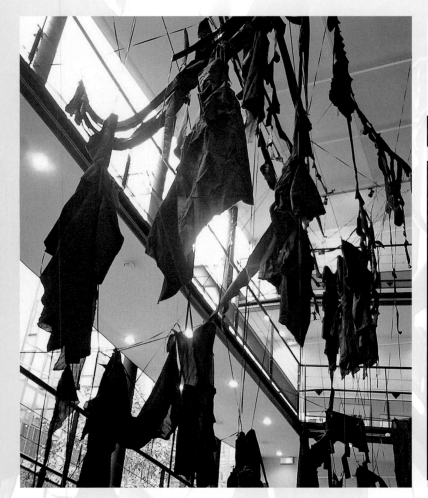

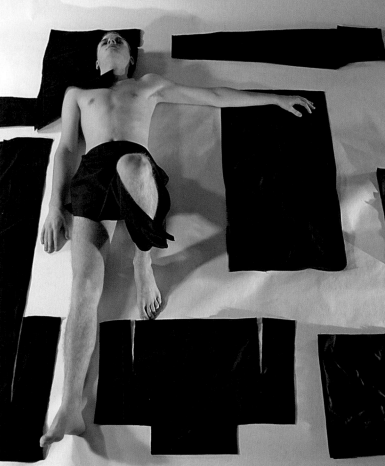

Joel Andrianomearisoa (Madagascar/ France) studied fashion in Madagascar before moving to Paris to study architecture. His approach to clothing design, which he describes as archi-couture, combines both of these influences. Adrianomearisoa often wraps his models in geometric shapes – they are sometimes made of fabric, but can also be rendered from other materials such as wood, stone and plastic. Rejection of French tailored clothing became a feature of Madagascan funerary ceremonies during the move for political independence. In Sakalava mortuary rites as well the bodies of Madagascan kings were wrapped in diverse coverings and enclosures.

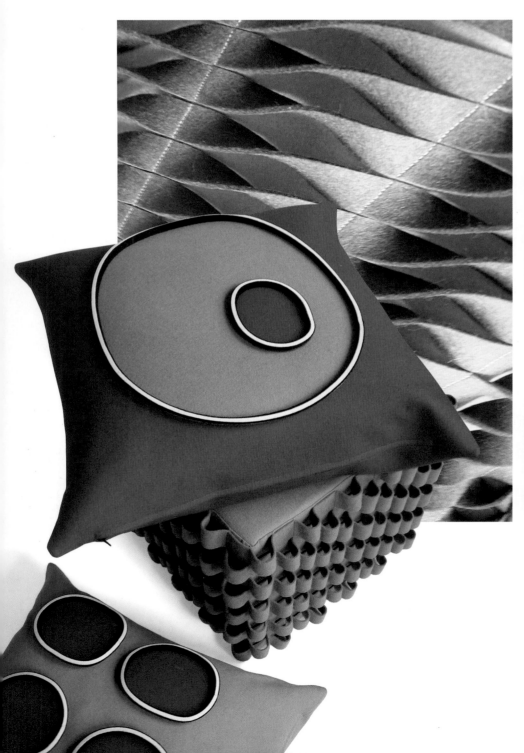

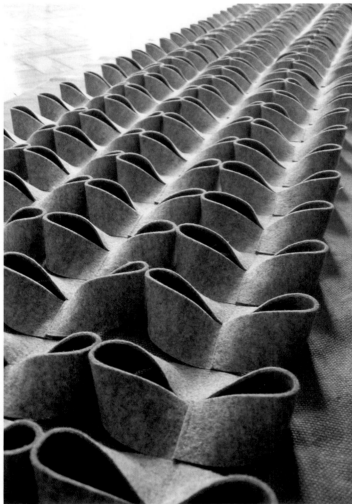

Anne Kyyrö Quinn (Finland), *Leaf* (2004),
stitched felt, *Target* (2003), stitched felt and linen,
and *Pod* (2004), stitched felt. London-based
Finnish designer Kyyrö Quinn uses felt, one of
the oldest fabrics known to mankind, to make
modernist, sculptural fabrics. *Target*, a
combination of appliqué and raised stitched
relief, is a fine example of the organic and
curvilinear forms that have become an
established feature of Scandinavian modernism.

Galya Rosenfeld (USA), *Multicolored, Modular Series*, 2002.

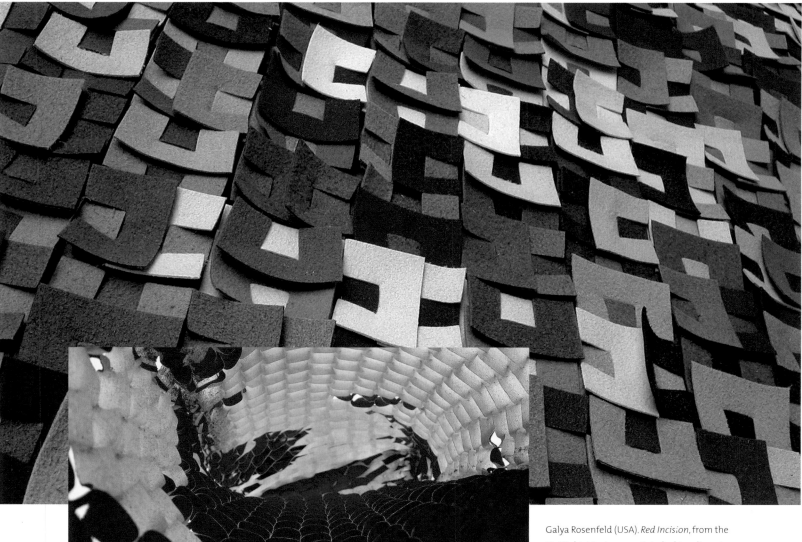

Galya Rosenfeld (USA). *Red Incision*, from the *Cut T-shirt Series*, 2003. Interlocking die-cut tab and slot modules are a way of making versatile cloths that can be slotted together. Dresses, shoes, bags, scarves and wall hangings made from remnants of rubber and synthetic suede can all be assembled without seams and can be adjusted to fit different circumstances. This close up is of a laser-cut T-shirt.

Lauren Moriarty (UK), *Noodle Block Cushion* (2006). Moriarty's lace cushions are laser cut from 2 mm thick sheets of neoprene before being heat-bonded into cushions. They are characteristic of her three-dimensional approach to textile design.

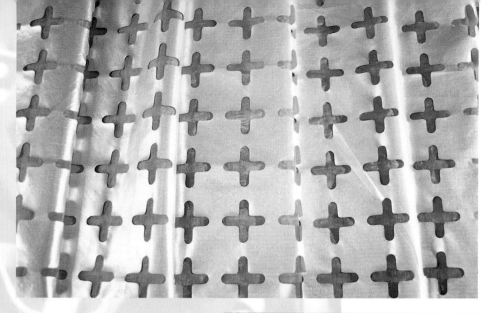

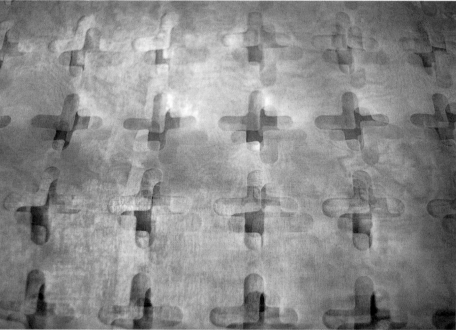

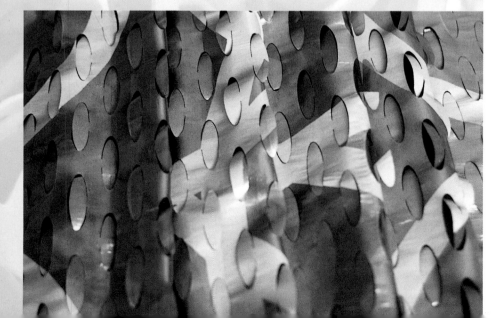

Leo Santos-Shaw (UK) and Margrét
Adolfsdóttir (Iceland) set up Santos +
Adolfsdóttir and create bespoke fabrics to
commission. Here, laser-cut and dyed
polyester and polyamide are superimposed
on top of a silk backing.

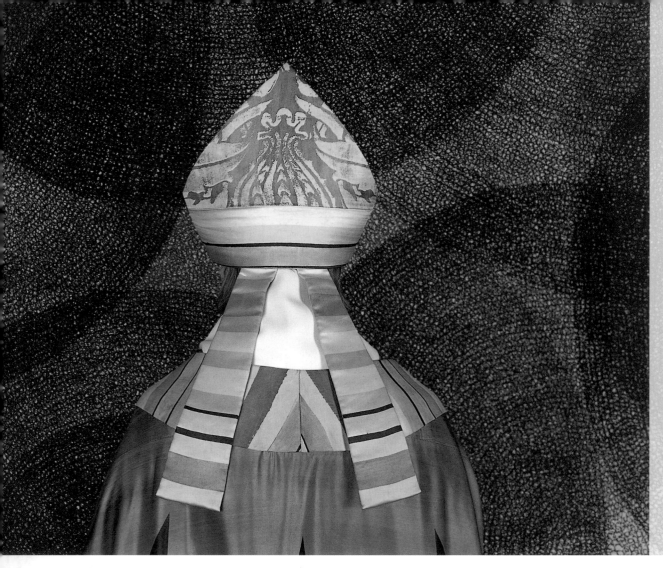

Victoria Richards (UK), *Discharge printed ecclesiastical robes* (2003).

In 2005 the modernist Milanese designer Nanni Strada began to design a contemporary chasuble (casula). Throughout her career Strada has researched ways of making clothes that circumvent Western tailoring, or which are better suited to a life of travel and movement: she became interested in the flat geometry of Japanese clothing in the 1960s and pioneered crinkle pleated travel clothes in the mid-1980s. Her interest in the chasuble is an extension of these concerns. Early members of the Christian church lived, slept and worshipped in these protective garments. Her aim was to convey the inner luminosity of the immaterial self by exploiting contemporary techniques of textile production. Strada's choice of materials permits a certain fluidity of gesture. The outer layer is made of satin which is perforated with laser-cut incisions, revealing glimpses of a luminous laminated satin undercoat beneath, rendered in the different colours of the liturgical year. Strada worked hard to achieve the 'deadened brilliance' she was looking for, persuading the silk manufacturer to process the laminated satin by adjusting the speed of the calendaring cylinders and modifying the heat-finishing process.

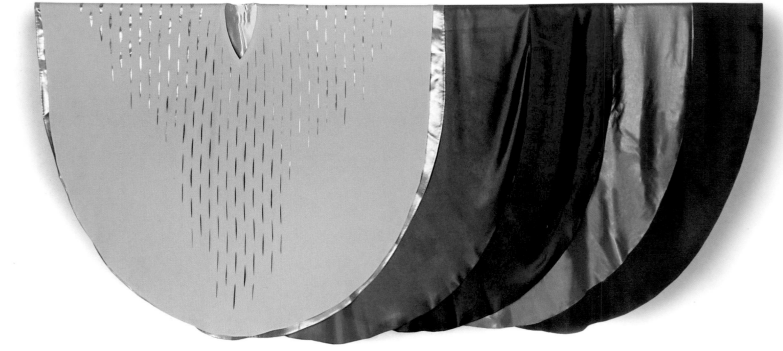

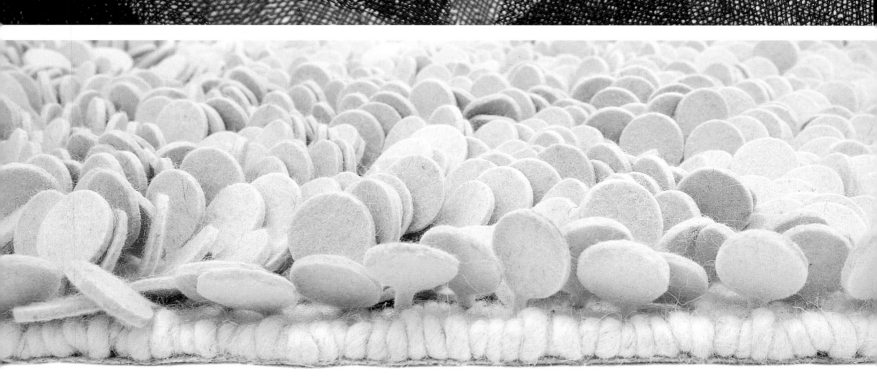

Aurora Caresi (Italy), *Layered wool felt* (2004).

Nani Marquina (Spain), *Roses* (2005). Hand-woven wool and felt.

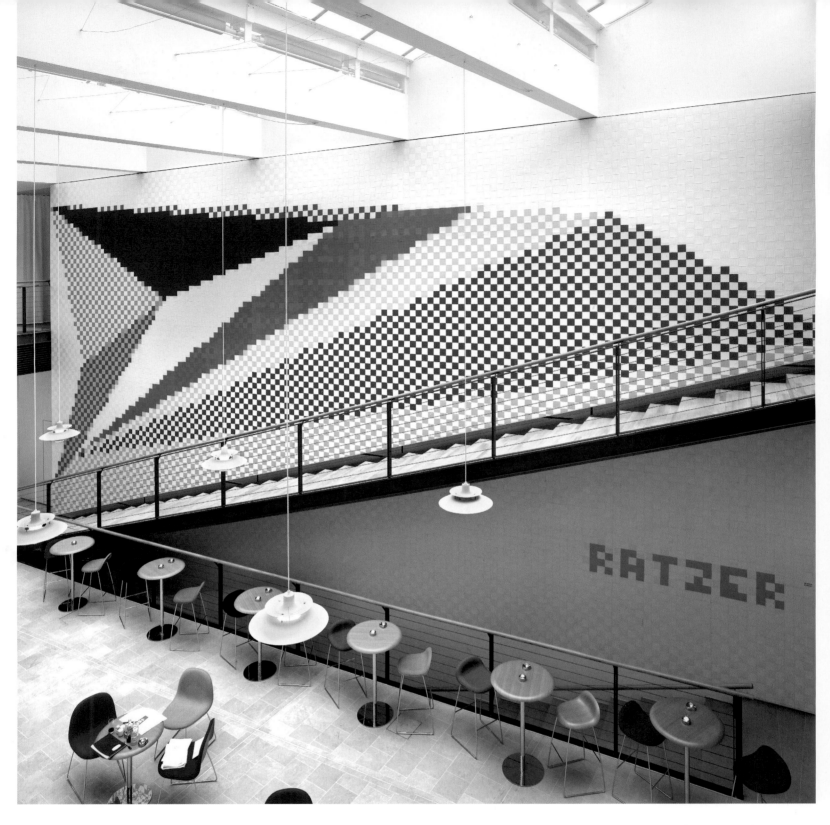

This wall hanging was made by Tina Ratzer (Denmark) from strips of cotton fabric woven onto a giant stretcher; it was commissioned by the Danish Design Centre in 2004. It is characteristic of Ratzer's three-dimensional approach to pattern perception. The abstract design shifts as it is viewed from different angles, exploiting the fact that visitors entering the room will initially be forced to view the pattern at an oblique angle, before they can see the design in its entirety.

Tina Ratzer, *Blossoming*, 2004 (opposite, above, right). Patchworked cotton made from floral prints found in a flea market combined with strips of cotton woven on a stretcher is a formal experiment in the scaling of pattern.

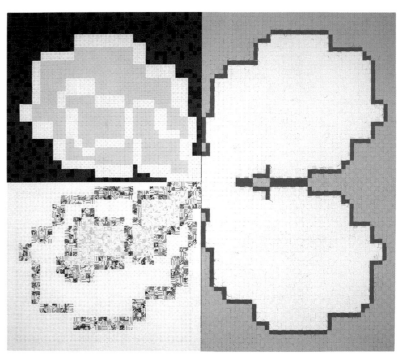

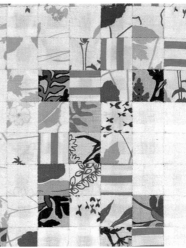

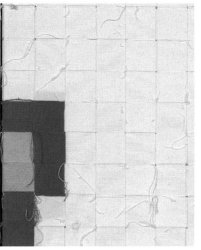

Two recent projects from Denmark show how textile designers are beginning to explore innovatively the way pattern is perceived in a specific architectural space. Danish designer Tina Ratzer's wall hanging for the Danish Design Centre (2004) is site specific. The complex, tessellated pattern made from plaited strips of cloth is an enlarged motif; the spatial form responds to the way that the visitor has to move through the space in which it hangs. Like the famous *memento mori* at the base of Hans Holbein the Younger's *The Ambassadors* (1533), Ratzer's wall hanging is an example of anamorphosis. This means that the formal arrangement of the pattern on the wall hanging appears to adopt different configurations when the visitor views it from an oblique angle – as indeed they move down the stairs flanking the work and into the hall.

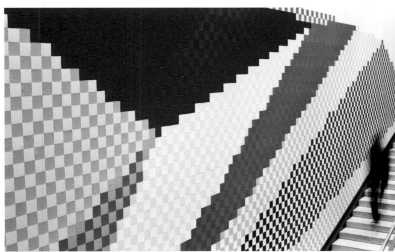

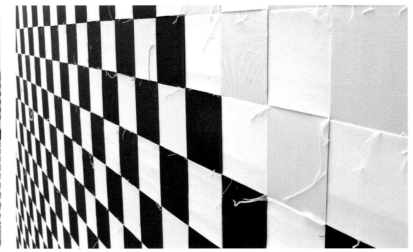

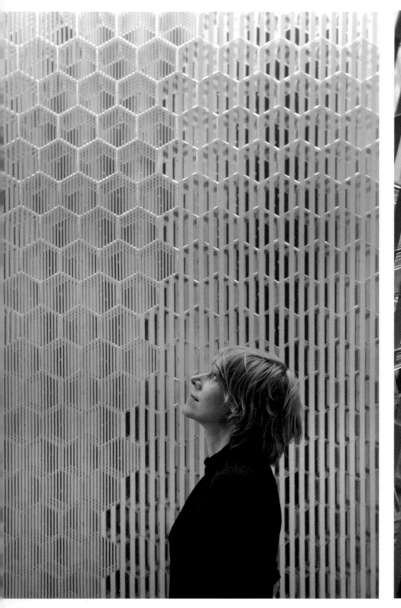

The way that the movement of the spectator modifies pattern perception was the subject of a recent exhibition at the Danish Design Centre. *Mind the Gap* (2006) was an installation mounted by Danish textile designer Ane Lykke. She covered the back wall of the room with two separate layers composed of hexagonal plastic boxes fitted with red stripes of varying density. These two layers create a form of interference, turning into large pattern areas that change with the light and the spectator's movements. As Lykke puts it, the wall is activated by the spectators' movements and by changes in light to form a living, vibrating surface. She explains:

'The exhibition explores a very common phenomenon, which we have all experienced, for example when passing two parallel grid fences. As we move we see new wave forms or patterns arising. "I want to find new ways of affecting the perception of a space, demonstrating that the spectator plays a crucial part."' Lykke points out that in physics this phenomenon is referred to as interference patterns.

Ane Lykke (Denmark), *Mind the Gap*, 2006. A pattern installation commissioned by the Danish Design Centre. One aspect of increasing interest in pattern perception has been the growth of popularity of interference patterns. Here Lykke has created a double wall of transparent perspex boxes embellished with stripes of varying widths. As visitors move around the room, the stripes appear to move relative to one another and create shifting, large-scale moiré images.

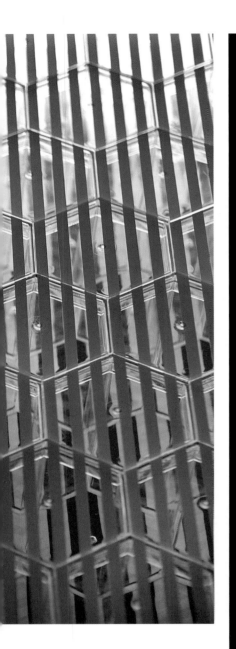

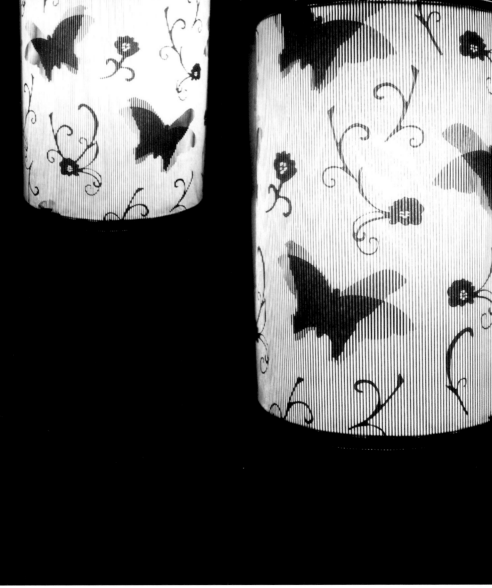

Lauren Moriarty (UK), *Butterfly Effect Lamp*, 2005, uses vertical stripes characteristic of lenticular imagery. The cylindrical shade combines two layers of pattern screen printed onto plastic to create an optical illusion. By layering patterns, Moriarty creates an interference effect that makes the butterflies' wings appear to flutter as you move around the room: if you stop moving, the butterfly stops too.

The Edge of Chaos, Pattern Formation and Error

The upsurge of interest in pattern formation in the natural sciences has been a great stimulus to many textile designers and artists. One of the more intractable issues it raises for designers and artists is to what extent such natural phenomena can be mitigated by free will or by individual decisions. The text-based work of the American textile artist Linda Hutchins uses the graphic form of words to explore the relationship between pattern formation in nature and the role of repetition in forming social preconceptions.

Hutchins' recent work is about the patterns that emerge when words are repeatedly typed on lengths of cloth or paper. The words are the kind of things that are said again and again: the admonitions repeated to children, 'be careful!', 'hurry up!', 'pay attention!', or the female virtues believed to be necessary for a happy married life, 'generosity, devotion, innocence'. Repeated on the typewriter, the shape of the letters and the intervals between the words make patterns as the lines continue down the lengths of cloth and paper – suggesting another dimension beyond the sense of the words themselves.

Hutchins has confessed an interest in catastrophe theory – a model used by natural scientists to understand how natural systems respond to disturbance. By applying these ideas to her type-written mantras, her work explores the way that chance upsets the

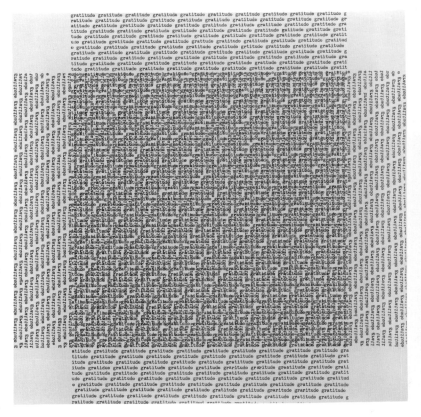

predictability of pattern – and by association the predictability of life. Some patterns emerge from type errors that inevitably occur as the artist types the same words repeatedly, others from odd breaks of text. Given a large enough field, such mistakes tend to repeat themselves, creating a new level of pattern. In one of her most ominous pieces of work, the phrase, 'You do not miss the water...until the well runs dry' meanders down lengths of cloth – the elaboration of a series of errors making the words resemble the kinds of rock strata through which the wells would be dug.

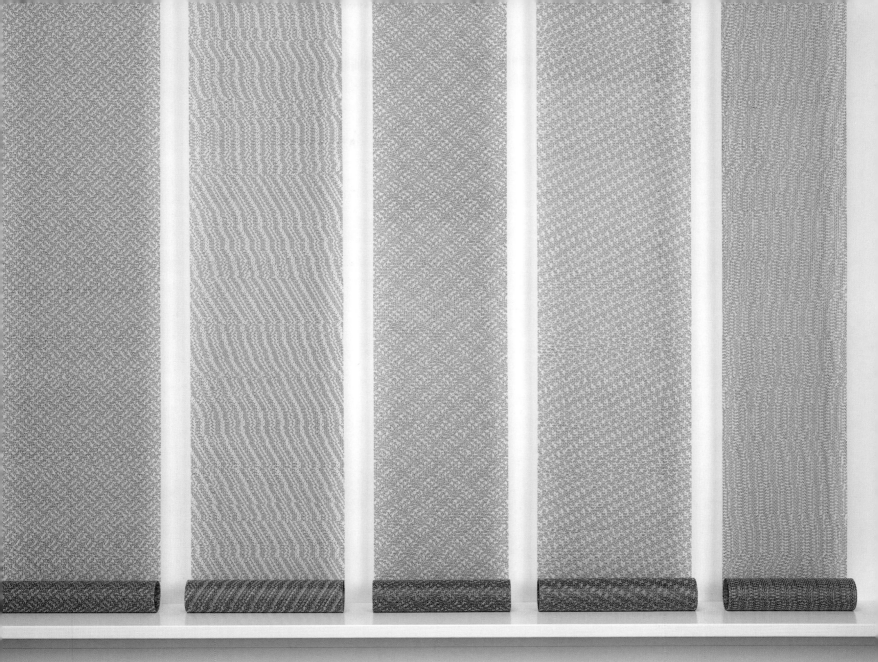

Linda Hutchins (USA), *Trousseau*, 2003 (detail), typewriting on twenty silk handkerchiefs that records the twenty different qualities desirable in a bride, and *Reiteration* (2003), typewriting on nine scrolls of vellum. *Reiteration* is a series of patterned images produced by repeatedly typing words and phrases on an old-fashioned typewriter. They are reminiscent of the work produced by the tormented character Jack Torrance in Stanley Kubrick's film, *The Shining* (1980); his madness becomes apparent when it is revealed that the manuscript he has been working on consists only of the repetitions and permutations of a single sentence. In Hutchins' hands these formal permutations are intricately elaborated to create beautiful, complex, lace-like patterns or moiré effects. Sometimes she types on both sides of a piece of fabric, in other instances patterns emerge from type errors and odd breaks in the text.

Hutchins' background is in computer engineering: she used to write systems software for Intel. Her work fuelled an interest in catastrophe theory, which demonstrates how small peripheral changes can upset the equilibrium of a complex geometric system, leading to fundamental changes of the system as a whole. In these typewritten pieces, the formal characteristics of pattern play off against her choice of message: the admonitions a parent makes to a child, warnings about care for the environment, suggesting that a latent threat, or tipping point, is imminent.

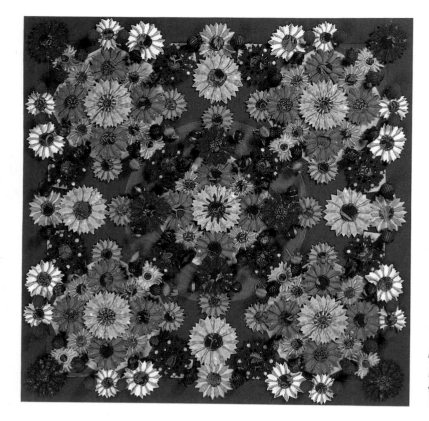

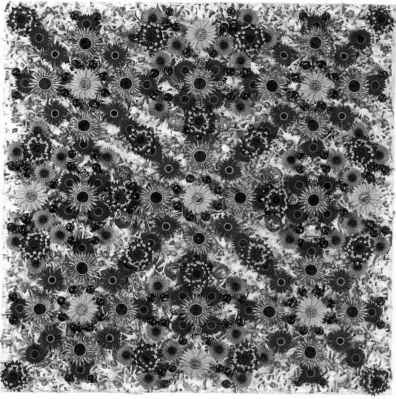

Across the natural sciences computer data are changing the way complex systems (that is, everything from ecological phenomena to biochemistry) are studied and arouse growing interest in pattern formation. Studies of pattern formation in fluid dynamics, which seek to understand the forms of waves, or the spontaneous, perfectly ordered pattern that water assumes as it splashes up in response to an object dropped into it, for example, are challenging 19th-century ideas about pattern resembling a language that evolves slowly and unconsciously over extended periods of time.

There is now growing interest in the way that life-like patterns emerge from a few relatively simple rules of interaction to achieve a precarious, and therefore dynamic, balance between chaos and order. British knitwear artist Freddie Robbins has put these ideas to work in a piece called *How to Make a Piece of Work When You Are Too Tired to Make Decisions* where all the main decisions regarding choice of yarn,

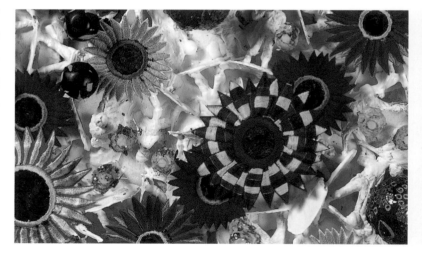

stitch and when to cast off have been made by the throw of a dice. The Icelandic textile artist Hildur Bjarnadóttir's drawings of Will Rogers's lasso work provide an example of the way that people are beginning to think of pattern in terms of movement.

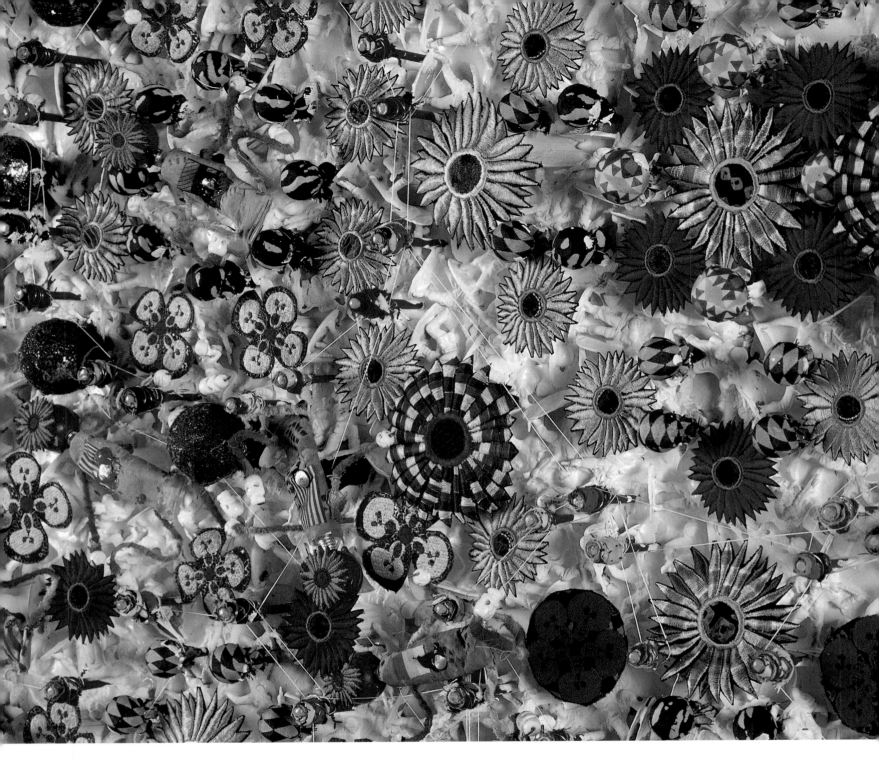

Michael Brennand-Wood (UK), *Consequence of Proximities – Walls Within Walls*, 2003 (opposite, left), *Crystallized Movements*, 2004 (opposite, above, right and detail) and *Died Pretty – Flag of Convenience*, 2005 (above). Brennand-Wood became one of the UK's leading textile artists during the mid-1980s. His new collection of work is a systematic investigation of the way that colour affects the formal structure of pattern. All his optical experiments are target-shaped and raise questions about the nature of vision. Brilliantly coloured machine-embroidered flowers, beads and other components are carefully positioned relative to one another to explore different permutations of emphasis within the same basic design. The titles are playful and the strident surface patterns are so strong that it is actually impossible to see through the surface of the design. In *Crystallized Movements* (2004), the target form becomes a representational device as striped flowers, reminiscent of medal ribbons, are layered on top of plastic soldiers.

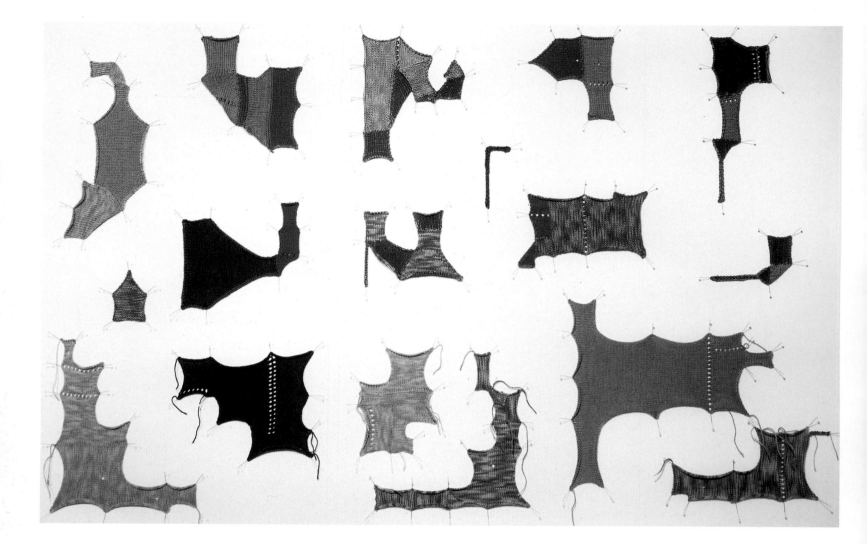

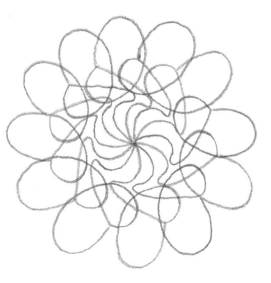

Freddie Robins (UK), *How to Make a Piece of Work When You Are Too Tired to Make Decisions* (2004) (above and opposite, above). Machine-knitted yarn, mounted on canvas. In Luke Rhinehart's 1972 cult book *The Dice Man*, the protagonist relinquishes moral responsibility by determining his actions with the throw of a dice. Robins, who is better known for her complex, machine-knitted sculptures that require a fine degree of mathematical calculation to work, applied the diceman's principles in this case to explore the relation between random design and pattern formation.

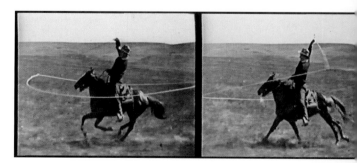

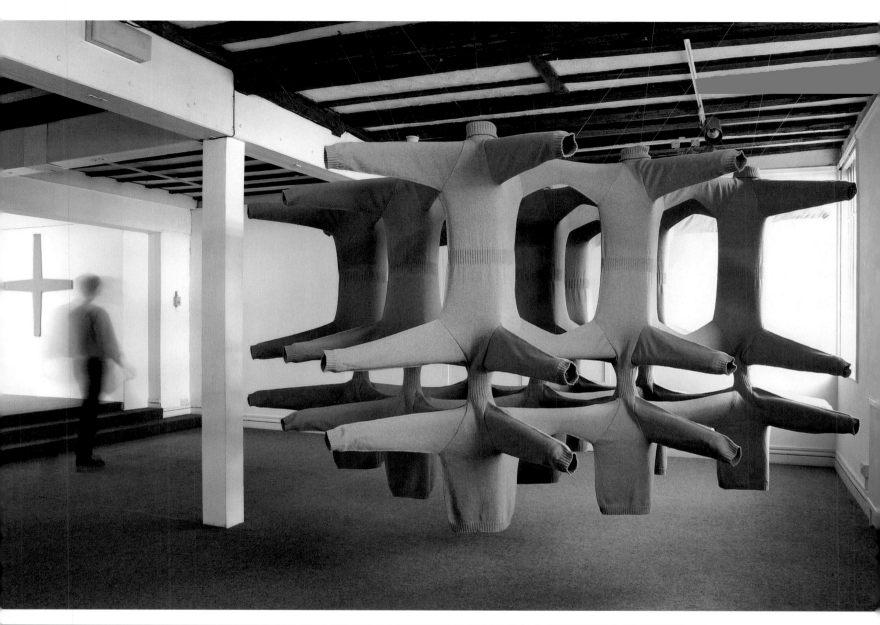

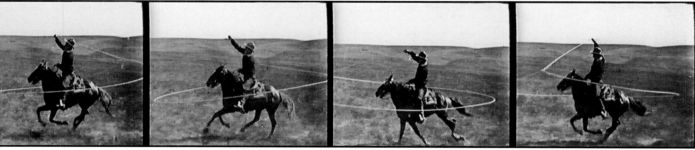

Icelandic textile artist Hildur Bjarnadóttir is best known for her work with tatting: a sturdy kind of lace made by looping and knotting thread, thought to have possibly been developed by sailors skilled in rope work. Her interest in the celebrated American lasso artist, Will Rogers, is a natural extension of this. Pictured here is a still from Rogers's celebrated silent movie *The Ropin' Fool* (1922), alongside Bjarnadóttir's schematic drawings of lasso motion.

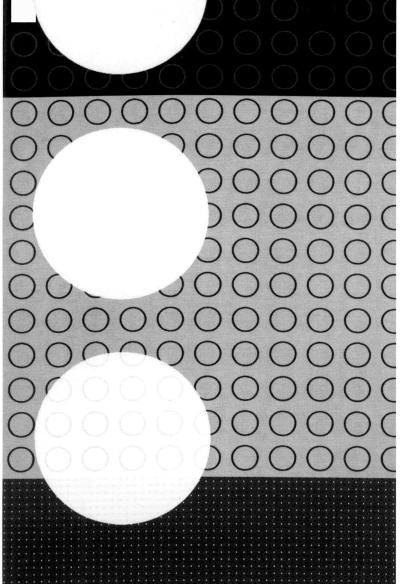

Hella Jongerius (Netherlands), *Repeat Dot* (2002), jacquard woven and screen-printed fabric. Jongerius is a conceptual, postmodern designer whose working method is to avoid designing new forms or patterns, but who aims to add a new dimension to the pre-existing patterns and forms she works with. Manufactured by Maharam, New York.

Hella Jongerius (Netherlands), *Repeat Classic* (2002), cotton, rayon and polyester jacquard weave. *Repeat*, which was commissioned by Maharam in New York to mark the company's centennial year, is characteristic of her meta-level approach to design : it is a pattern about pattern repetition across intervals of space and time. The scale of the repeat presents a way of producing a form of kinship from a mass-produced fabric, since it is highly improbable that identical pieces of furniture will feature the same section of pattern. All of the pattern elements were taken from Maharam's archives.

The Dutch designers Hella Jongerius and Tord Boontje have both shown an interest in incorporating random error into the design of factory-made objects as a way of imbuing them with the character that makes people attached to hand-made objects. In the work of these two designers giving way to serendipity is married to a hands-off approach towards form; this may explain why Chaos theory has appealed to post-modernist designers. Both Jongerius and Boontje explored these issues during the 1990s, while working for Droog, the experimental Dutch design collaborative, where they applied these ideas to a range of different fields of design. Jongerius, for example, has worked with equal success in areas of design that have traditionally been male-dominated such as furniture design, as well as areas of decorative design such as ceramics and textiles where women have predominated, but which have traditionally been regarded as marginal. 'The reason that I work in [ceramics and textiles]', she recently explained in an interview, 'is because I can add a lot of layers. Function is minimal so you can play about using strange combinations of techniques, or add historical things to a contemporary language.'

Jongerius has recently worked to commission for Chicago-based upholstery manufacturer Maharam, which has an established reputation for well-designed office furnishing fabrics. In her design Jongerius used compilations of motifs from Maharam's archives of jacquard cloth

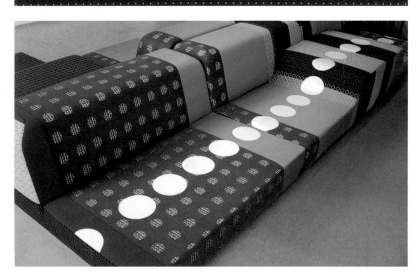

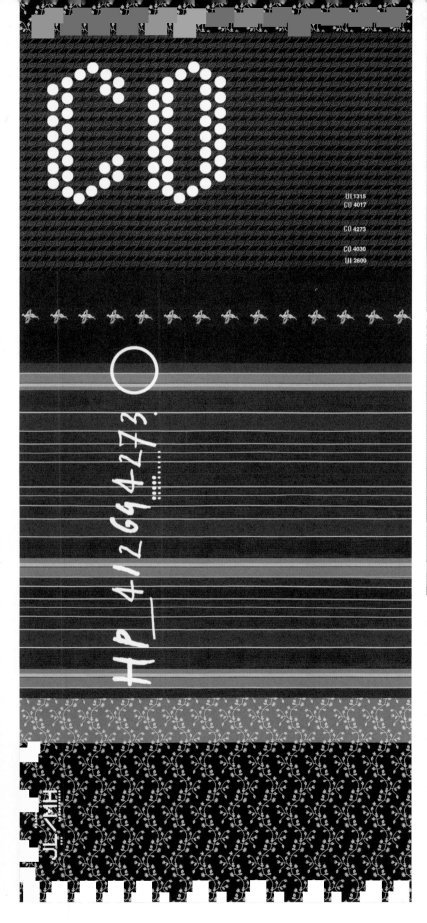

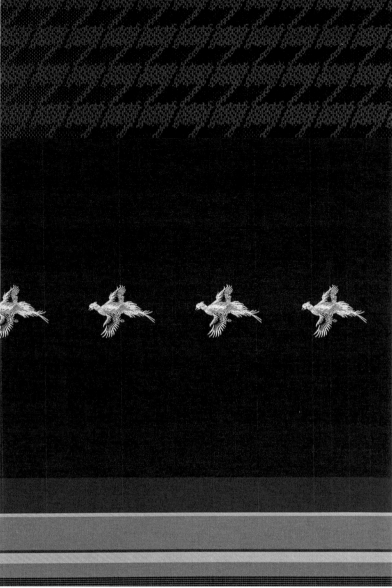

to create a new series of woven and printed fabrics. Here the 'mistake' was to make the patterns huge (each repeat is three metres wide) and so inevitably out of scale with individual pieces of furniture so that the pattern has to spill from one piece to the next, creating the possibility for random effects. The pattern is overprinted with codes from jacquard punch cards and hand-written pattern codes: the kind of behind-the-scenes technical information that is usually kept out of sight. It is this deliberate wrong-footedness that helps to provoke a more thoughtful and considered approach to pattern.

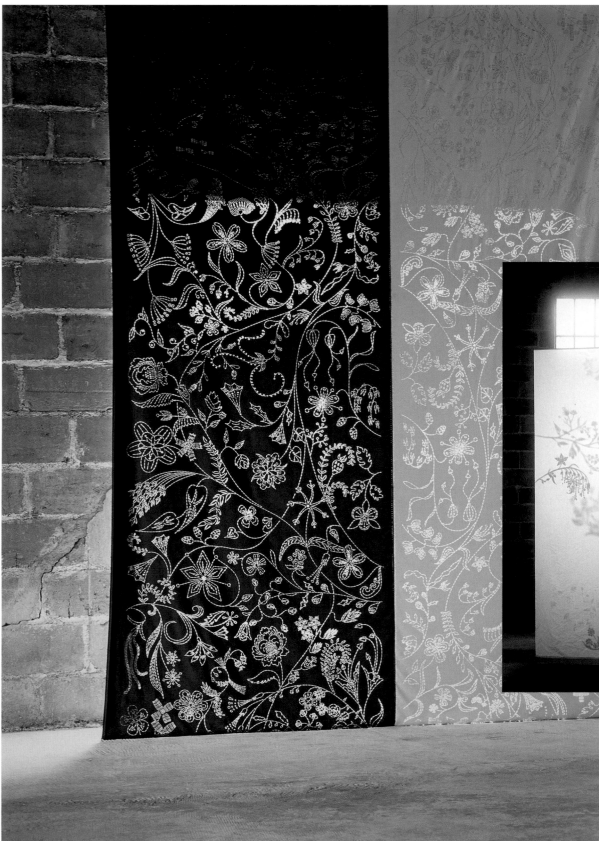

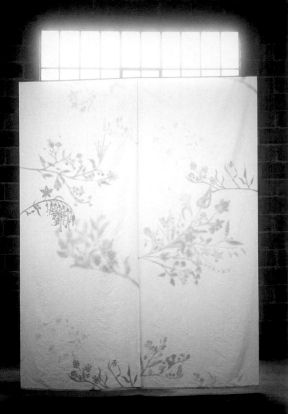

In 2003 Bruce Stirling named Tord Boontje as a key exponent of Tech Nouveau, seeing in his work a modern interpretation of the sinuous tendrils and luxuriant flowers and foliage of the Art Nouveau style. Whether people adopt this label, or another, such as 'organic minimalism' (which acknowledges the influence of the 1960s revival of Art Nouveau upon the current interpretation), the popularity of Boontje's romantic floral patterns seems to many to confirm that we are entering a new era of pattern aesthetics. Laser cutting has inspired much of Boontje's pattern work. In his case, this technology has provoked an interest in silhouettes and in folk traditions of paper cutting.

Tord Boontje (Netherlands), *Eternal Summer* (2005) (above) is a laser-cut blackout curtain, manufactured by Kvadrat, Denmark. The design is seen at its best when daylight shines through the perforations, casting an illuminated floral pattern on the floor and walls.

Boontje has also relinquished a degree of the control of form in order to convey the way patterns move and evolve. In a recent project called Inflorescence, which was developed with Andrew Shoben from the digital art collaborative, Grey World, and the computer programmer Andrew Allenson, Boontje developed a computer-animated pattern in which flowers could be seen to bud, grow and decay, and even showed their dying petals being blown across the screen. The programme draws flower patterns in a random manner and it draws them differently each time, forgetting what it has done before. It is the flexibility of digital design, Boontje argues, that has enabled designers to develop a new interest in 17th-, 18th- and 19th-century decorative art, in place of the stark forms of modern design. Boontje envisaged the programme being used directly to generate subtly differentiated outputs in the form of embroidery, printing, etching or computer lithography.

These examples all show how designers are beginning to open up the design process with an element of chance. Nevertheless, there is also something frightening about the way that digital media can produce forms of artificial life that not only replicate, but also evolve in a manner that is detached from subjective observation.

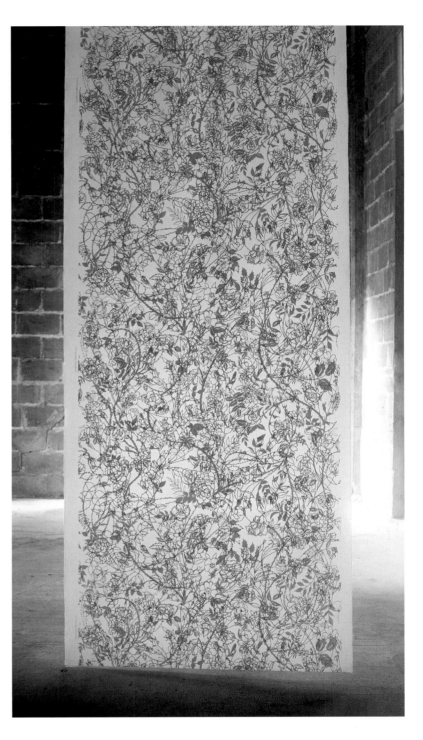

Tord Boontje (Netherlands), *The Pattern of Shadow* (2005) (opposite, left) is digitally printed and ebbs and fades across the surface of the polyester net curtain, casting a fluid wash of shadow on the floor.

Tord Boontje (Netherlands), *Sleeping Rose* (2005), manufactured by Kvadrat, Denmark. By overlapping two versions of this floral pattern on top of each other, *Sleeping Rose* suggests a protective thicket of bramble and briar rose.

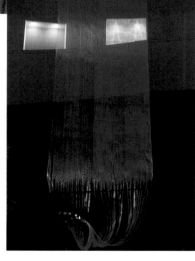

Astrid Krogh (Denmark), *Holbein Neon Tapestry* (2002). A light weaving made from optical fibre. Plastic fibre optics are now flexible enough to be woven on the loom. In this piece the ends of the fibres are connected to a computer monitor which radiates colour to light up them.

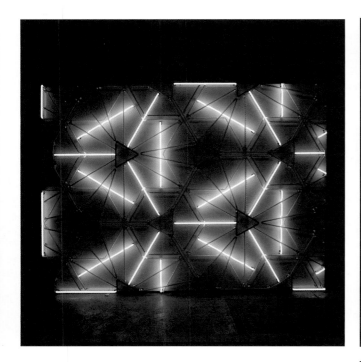

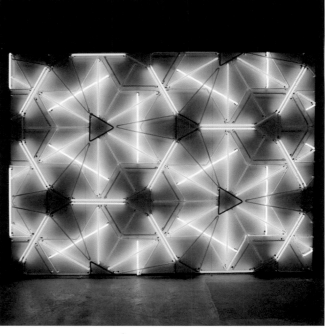

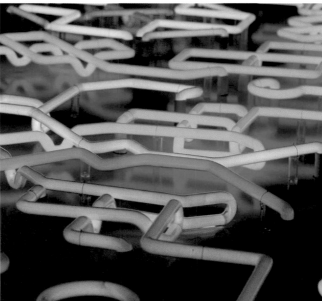

Astrid Krogh (Denmark), *Ornament Neon Wallpaper* (2003) is a study in pattern variation. 186 neon lights are arranged in ten sections and can be combined in different ways to generate over 3 million different pattern variations.

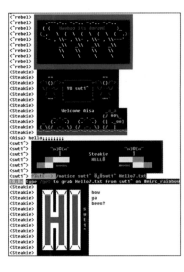

Pattern, Textiles and Digital Interaction

A concern with conveying the particularity of urban environments in different parts of the world may have also been fuelled by anxiety about the nature of digital culture: the fear that experience in cyberspace is in some way disembodied from physical experience or isolated from the real world and our normal attachments – to place, to profession, to religious denomination or ethnic affiliation – that make up our grounded identities. According to this view, an internet chat room would be the polar opposite of the independent design studios where many of the designers mentioned in this chapter conduct their work. Yet chat rooms do have the advantage of boosting social interaction, which provokes a way of working that is quite distinct from individualist studio practice.

At a grassroots level, Windows 95 has provided both a social medium as well as a set of graphic tools of expression that has led to the rapid development of new way of working in pattern. The participants of #mIRC_Rainbow, a channel of Microsoft's Internet Relay Chat (IRC, one of the world's most popular internet chat rooms) have used the letters and typographic symbols of the computer keyboard to create patterns and imagery. The kind of chat that takes place on #mIRC_ Rainbow is distinct because the participants' exchanges are predomi-nantly image based and unlike most ASCII artists, whose work is mono-chrome, their work shows a love of pattern and colour. To a certain extent, Rainbow artists seemed to enjoy the degree of anonymity that the IRC chatroom afforded them. Most used computer 'nicks' (nick-names) and though many had their own websites, it was unusual for these to feature any direct clues as to the participant's home address, so it took some investigating to establish that the majority of the devoted friends were from the American South or the Mid West. Yet Professor Brenda Danet from Yale University, who made an ethnographic study of the chat room between 1997 and 2002, monitored the tens of thou-sands of patterned and ornamented messages that were exchanged during this period and reached the surprising conclusion that far from encouraging social atomization, IRC provided the perfect conditions for the accelerated emergence of a new kind of folk art.

Despite a high turnover of visitors, many of the hundred or so devoted friends of #mIRC_Rainbow were interested in real world crafts and in textile crafts such as quilting or embroidery in particular. This meant that although the patterns were strictly ephemeral – i.e., they could only be viewed when the participant was logged on and connected to an IRC channel – there was a latent material dimension to them nevertheless. Another important point was that although most of Rainbow participants never met face to face, the emphasis on real-time

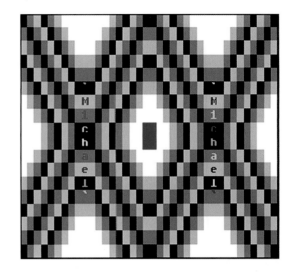

interaction enforced certain social conventions. New participants (newbies) were typically assigned operatives who taught them how to manipulate imagery according to certain rules in a process very similar to a classic apprenticeship. An ethos of sharing became established very quickly which meant that the creators of new images were expected to include guidelines about how to download patches from their own design. Furthermore, although many of the patterns were generic and even derivative, since many images were taken from existing collections of ASCII art and figurative images tended to draw upon shared imagery, there were, in fact, quite complex rules of etiquette regarding the acknowledgement of ASCII artists' work.

The combination of communications technology and textiles can also suggest other paths of creativity, which are at once local and international in character. Information networks have provoked the revival of low-tech forms of popular craft such as hand knitting. Not so long ago hand knitting was a relatively homely activity. Skilled knitters earned the respect of their immediate family and perhaps their local community, but were essentially unknown outside these spheres. The 1980s saw the rise of celebrity knitting designers such as Kaffe Fassett and today, the key protagonists in the world of knitting have become celebrity amateurs in the increasingly internet-based world of knitting

groups. They attend knitting conventions, festivals and happenings at rock concerts or in parks and other public venues in the United States, Europe, Japan and Australia, and they sustain a community of followers through their written commentary and exchange of opinion about these activities in the form of blogs and conversations conveyed through IRC.

Many club participants see knitting as a way of marking their distance from global corporate culture. The objects made are playful and naïve – sometimes to the point of infantilism. The wool and the needles are oversize. Everyone agrees that this is primarily a social phenomenon – more about people and attitude and chat rather than the creative process. The internet has played a vital role in developing this social dimension. The names of the clubs, such as 'crafternoon', 'cittyknitty', and the nicknames of the web leaders such as 'knitwit', as well as the acronyms used in web chat, such as WIP (work in progress), UFO (unfinished object), or best of all, TOAD (trashed object, abandoned in disgust), all help to establish a gulf between the new clubs and the kind of serious skill-based approach to knitting espoused by the Women's Institute.

The craze for setting up regionally based knitting clubs has spread from the northern United States to Britain and Australia and there are

Dholli, Roll me over in the clover (1997–2003) #mIRC_Rainbow. Glide translation of an asymmetric figurative motif of seven clover flowers. The original ASCII motif is by Joan Stark. It is composed of typographic symbols and is rendered in a manner that is reminiscent of the stitching on a sampler. The name of the rainbow artist is unknown. Brenda Danet was interested to discover that many of the participants, who come largely from the American South and the Mid-West, had a real-world interest in craft textiles. She has argued that many of these exchanges should be seen as a kind of digital fabric.

A patterned greeting presented by Michael to one of the participants on his birthday in 1997 corroborates her point.

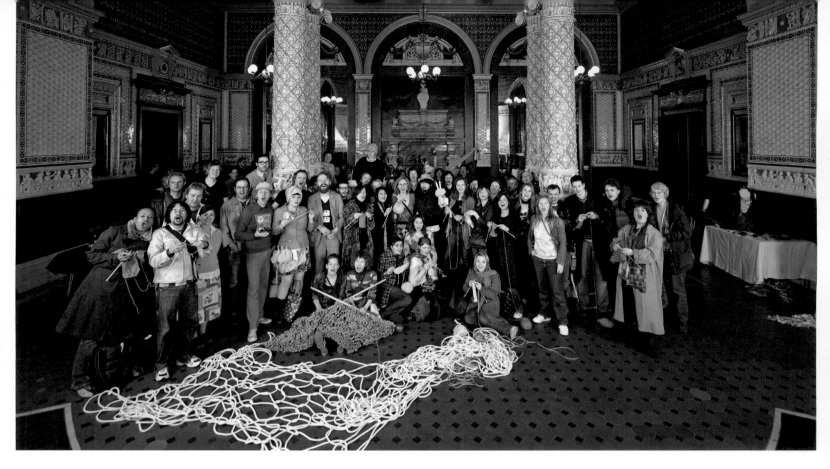

now several hundred of these clubs, making the movement both local-ized and international in character. It also links internet activity to the real world. Whereas Rainbow art is exclusively web based, KIP (knitting in public) is a vital dimension of most of the knitting clubs' activities, since the collective 'outing' of female craft in public is a shared concern. The London-based group Cast Off, which was started by Rachael Matthews in 2000, has organized events on the Circle Line of the tube, in pubs, at political rallies and even in the Savoy bar, from which they were thrown out, as well as the phenomenally successful Craft Rocks event at the Victoria and Albert Museum in London which attracted nearly 3,000 participants. It is a forceful reminder that the relationship between digital culture and real world events may be more complex than is first apparent.

Knitting groups are, of course, not directly connected with pattern *per se*, but they do show how the internet is regenerating interest in popular creativity. Such conditions are much more conducive to the appreciation of pattern than 20th-century models of top-down design, based upon modernist ideas of creativity and originality. It was during the 20th century that the capacity to make and recognize pattern came to be seen as something atavistic, a part of our cognitive makeup that had been hard wired within us during an earlier stage of our evolution. In the 21st century pattern seems to have found a place in contemporary civilized culture. It is surely no coincidence that, given the widening internet audience, and the increasingly multi-cultural character of cities around the world, pattern's capacity to capture the spatial character and references that inflect contemporary culture at a given point in time has begun to attract so much attention. Combined with the renewed interest in form and de-centred pattern formation in the natural sciences, it would seem that one of the primary features of textile aesthetics may at last be in a position to receive the attention it deserves.

SUN 2
JULY

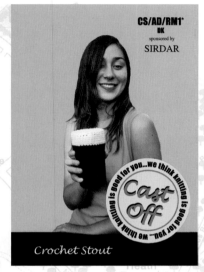

CS/AD/RM1*
DK
sponsored by
SIRDAR

Cast Off

Crochet Stout

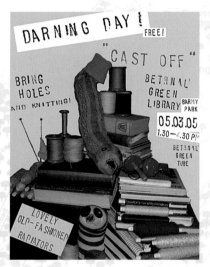

DARNING DAY !   FREE!
" CAST OFF "
BRING HOLES AND KNITTING!
BETHNAL GREEN LIBRARY   BARMY PARK
05.03.05
1.30 — 4.30 PM
BETHNAL GREEN TUBE
LOVELY OLD-FASHIONED RADIATORS

Cast Off, which bills itself as a knitting group for boys and girls, is an online knitting group that instigates public knitting events in parks, street fairs, on the underground and in nightclubs. Pictured here are the flyers circulated to invite participants to some of these events. In 2004 they curated Craft Rocks at the Victoria and Albert Museum, London, which attracted 2,873 visitors.

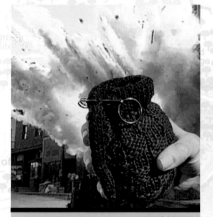

HKHG/ RRM/ 1
Hand Knitted
Hand Grenade!

It's also a purse! Drop stitches not bombs, with ' Cast Off ©

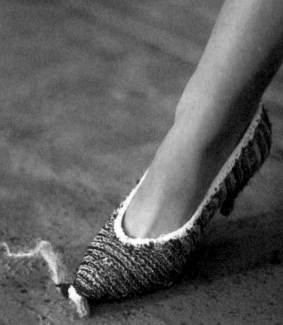

Cast Off,
knitting club for boys and girls.

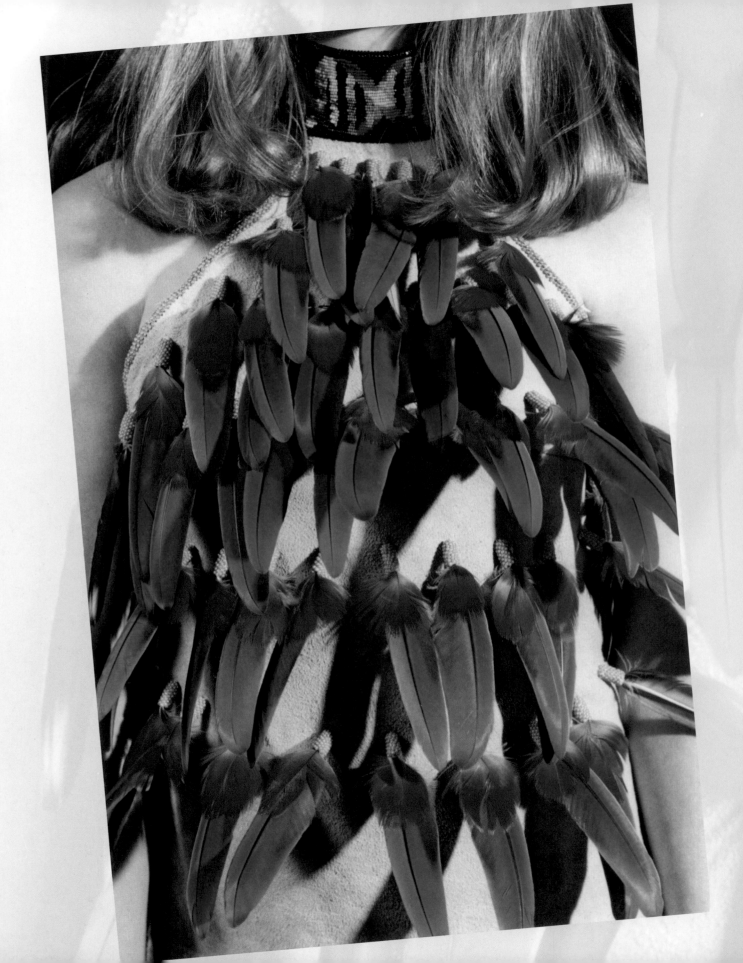

Textiles, Art and Culture

Over recent years interest in textiles among artists and academics has grown enormously. This interest has its roots in several different trajectories, coming from both inside and outside the art world. In the late 20th century people became interested in textiles because they extended beyond a local, Western system of classification for fine art. Textiles began to be valued because they were part of life, because they were central to the ceremonies marking the passage, or cycle of life, and because they were an important feature of so many non-Western artistic traditions. However, at the very point that textiles began to attract attention because they seemed offer a purchase on cultural diversity, people began to question the nature of culture conveyed by ethnographic exhibits and why it was that, in the case of textiles at least, museum exhibits differed so much from the hybrid fabrics and clothing styles encountered on the streets..

The view that useful, everyday objects could communicate important insights about the human condition was a recurrent theme of 20th-century art that had emerged through the work of Dadaists, Surrealists, conceptual artists and Pop artists, all of whom had challenged the orthodox view that insists upon the detachment of art from everyday life. In the latter part of the 20th century textiles also played a key part in the changes that took place in the contemporary art world as it expanded to involve work by increasing numbers of women as well as growing numbers of artists from different ethnic backgrounds. These changes meant that the use of cloth to invoke issues of cultural representation came to eclipse other, previously important

Marcus Amerman (USA), *DNA Dress*, 1999. Made of buckskin, size 13 cut beads and parrot feathers.

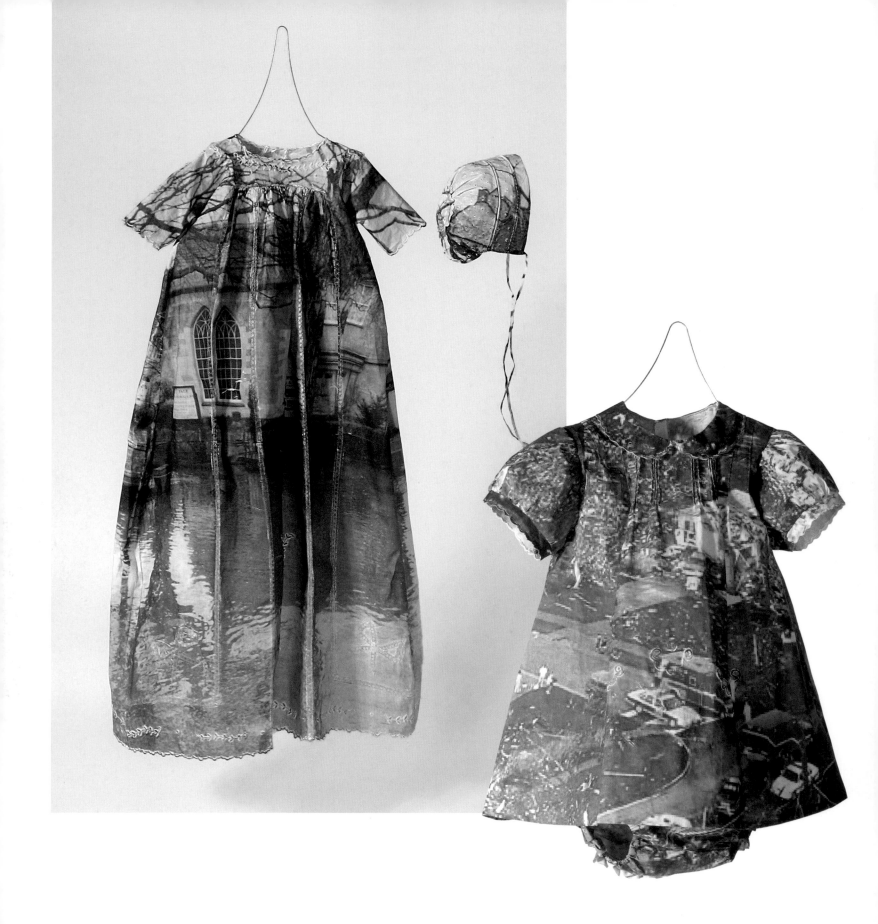

trajectories that had dominated European textile art hitherto: for instance, the transformation of the European aristocratic tradition of tapestry, or the development of folk art traditions such as quilting into a form of art in the United States, or the experiment with material, structure and figuration that had interested a previous generation of craft practitioners and textile artists.

In the 1970s a number of feminist artists began to work with 'female' decorative traditions such as embroidery, for example, instead of predominantly 'masculine' fine art media such as oil paint, metal and stone, in order to investigate the hidden histories of women's artistic expression outside established art-historical canon. At roughly the same time artists from different ethnic backgrounds started to look to local materials and their own artistic traditions in order to combat the cultural imposition of Eurocentric definitions of fine art upon them.

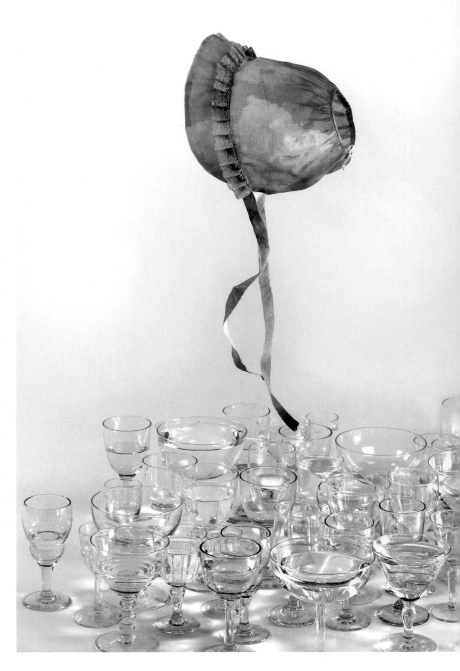

Shelly Goldsmith (UK), *Baptism*, 2003. A reclaimed christening gown that has been heat-transfer printed with a digitally adjusted photograph of recent flood damage in Britain. It is characteristic of her multi-layered vision of the use of resources.

The bell-shaped dress and pants were made by the employees of a children's home in Cincinnati and have been overprinted with digital images of a tornado that were taken by the Cincinnati Red Cross.

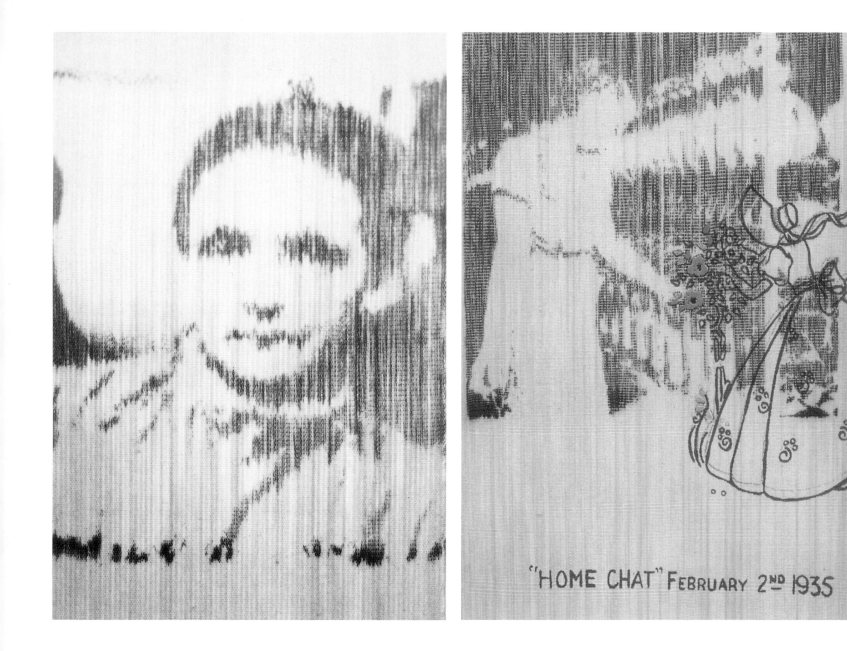

"HOME CHAT" FEBRUARY 2ND 1935

Julie Graves (UK), *Home Chat*, 1992. This warp-printed fabric featuring an image of a mill worker adjusting a loom is worked with a twee picture of a woman tending her garden from a standard embroidery kit; it reveals the gulf between the representation of femininity through embroidery and women's experience of working in the textile trade.

Textile Culture
and the Ethnographic Museum

Textiles have long been seen as a crucial source of information about other places and cultures and they figure prominently in anthropological collections, often referred to as 'ethnographic collections', which were built up during the 19th century by European colonialists. As collectable items, they have shaped our understanding of material culture – a category established through museum practice that selectively represents the heterogeneity of non-Western art traditions. Textile collections have generated their own specialist institutions of textile research and conservation, as well as of museum display. However, by the early 1990s many of these conventions of display and organization were criticized for perpetuating a false sense of division between modern and traditional cultures. Ethnographic collections were housed in separate buildings in museums of contemporary art and fostered a way of representing textiles – by treating them as scientific, natural specimens, or by classifying them according to region as opposed to historical period, for example – that exaggerated their distance from the history of commerce and largely overlooked the changes initiated during the colonial period. In fact, up until the late 1980s textiles from Africa, Oceania, the Americas and the remote communities of South-East Asia were valued for the perceived stability and isolation of the traditions they represented: an attitude to authenticity that persists at many collectors' fairs today.

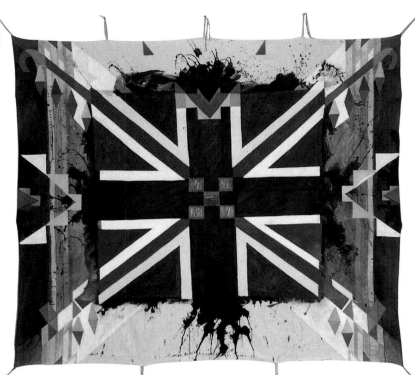

In the mid-1980s, when indigenous artists began to exhibit their work in contemporary art galleries many found textiles were a potent medium to explore the impact of European trade upon indigenous art. Native Canadian artist, Bob Boyer, for example, substituted canvas for Hudson Bay Blankets, goods used in European trade with Native Americans on the Plains that became notoriously linked to the spread of smallpox to the Native American population during the 19th century. *A Minor Sport in Canada* (1985) equates the violence of the European domination of Native Americans with the violence of cultural assimilation – a Union Jack is violently imposed on top of motifs characteristic of the Plains Native Americans, which ooze blood. More recently, another Native American artist, Marie Rose Watt, has used Hudson Bay Blankets and quilting to suggest that the necessary elements for cultural revival and renewal lie close to hand in the liminal sleep world that exists in parallel to waking life. Both she and Choctaw artist Marcus Amerman, who uses beadwork (another good that played a prominent part in the

Bob Boyer (Saskatchewan Indian Canadian), *A Minor Sport in Canada*, 1985, made from a blanket over painted with acrylic and oil paint, shows how textile trade goods could be used to explore colonial history. One of the *Blanket Statements* for which the artist became famous, this piece was inspired by an article that the artist read about the Battle of Batoche (1885), the culmination of the confrontation of the North-West Rebellion, which suggested that government troops viewed it as a sporting adventure. This image is courtesy of the National Gallery of Canada.

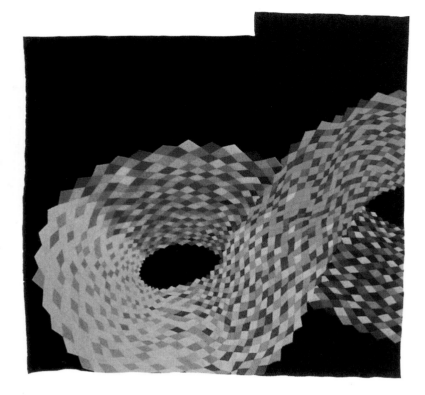

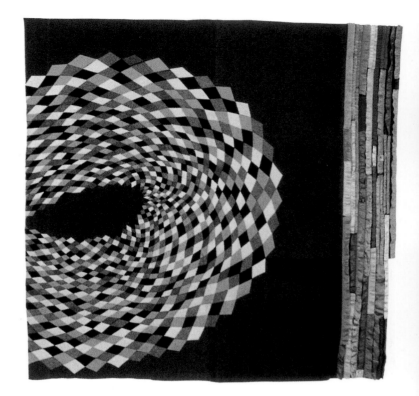

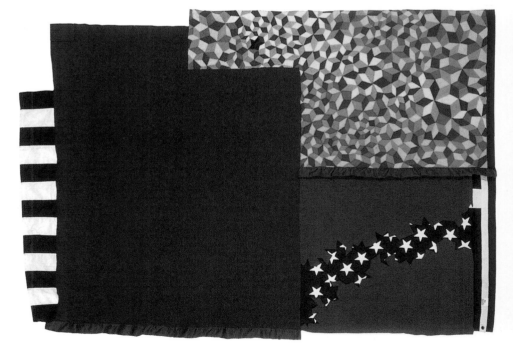

Marie Rose Watt (USA), *Braid*, 2004, reclaimed wool, satin binding, thread. The piece was completed with the help of 77 friends and family members who participated in sewing bees at the artist's studio.

Marie Rose Watt (USA), *Edson's Flag*, 2004. An American flag, passed down from the artist's uncle who served as an aeroplane mechanic during the Second World War, worked with appliquéd remnants of miscellaneous wool blankets as well as a Army, Navy and Hudson Bay trade blankets.

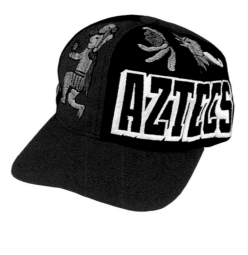
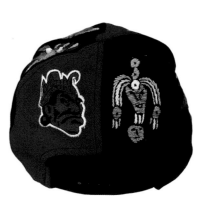

trade between the Native American and settler communities), convey contemporary aspects of Native American culture in order to challenge the static and conventional view of Native American art sustained by the demands of white collectors.

Nigerian-born British artist Yinka Shonibare has used African wax prints, a material that he found on the streets of Brixton in London, to address dimensions of the relationship between Britain and Africa that were not being made visible elsewhere. 'When I was at art college, I remember, I was doing a series of pieces about *perestroika*, which was a new kind of development in the Soviet Union at the time. And one of my tutors came up to me and said that "Ooh it's all right you're doing stuff about the Soviet Union, but it's not really you though is it?" And I thought… 'Okay, you want ethnic, I'll give you ethnic'. I kind of threw out all my canvases and I went to Brixton market, looking around as you do. And I started to think about the origins of *Ankara*, African fabric.'

African wax prints, roller-printed fabrics originally derived from Indonesian *batik* (called *Ankara* in Nigeria), are immensely popular and are worn by millions of people in sub-Saharan Africa today. A product of colonial, and more recently international trade, they bring together Africa, Europe, East Asia and elsewhere (the fabrics are now manufac-

tured in Malaysia and Pakistan). Dutch Wax fabric – resist-printed imitations of *batik* initially destined for colonial markets in Indonesia – was introduced by English merchants at the end of the 19th century to colonial markets in West Africa. Then in the 1920s roller-printed imitations were produced in Manchester for the same markets.

Initially Shonibare's work addressed the implications of using colonial cottons in the de-Westernization campaigns. These fabrics were a feature of the African independence movements of the 1960s, where Western-style dress was rejected in favour of flowing robes and dresses made from African wax prints produced in the new textile factories that were springing up throughout Western and Southern Africa during this period. This was a time when African prints 'became a symbol of nationalist revival in the wake of political independence in Africa, a sign of a new continent, of pride and difference': an optimism, Shonibare's work suggests, that was vulnerable from the outset. In *Cha cha cha* (1997), for example, a pair of women's stiletto shoes is presented in a riveted glass display case, like a museum exhibit. The shoes are covered with a design taken from a Dutch Wax pattern (many of which remain in circulation today), featuring the sole of a foot, a design that was formerly known in the textile trade by the pejorative name *nigger's footprint*.

Rubén Ortiz Torres (USA), customized baseball cap, 2001, showing his reinterpretation of the Aztec logo.

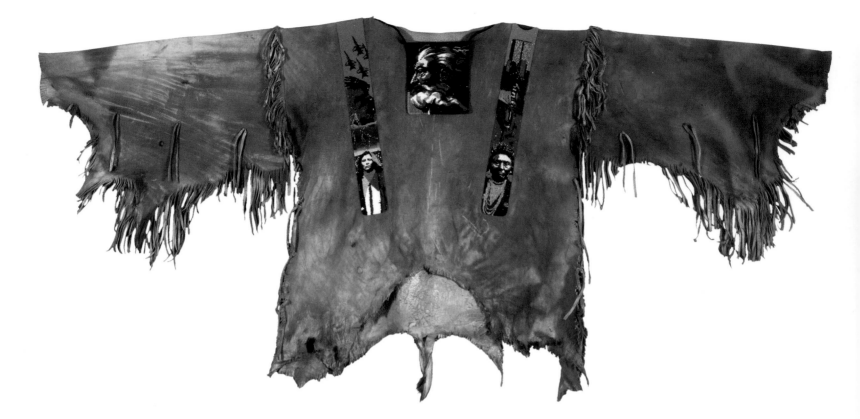

The title *Cha cha cha* is an oblique reference to President Mobutu's authenticity campaign during the Zairean independence movement of the mid-1960s (*Independence chacha* by Grand Kalle was the song that was played in bars across Kinshasa at the time and came to epitomize the optimism of the period). At this time Mobutu first started promoting Mobutu suits, or *abacos* (from the French 'à bas la costume' which means 'down with the suit'), complex garments that were cut in the style of a Chinese safari suit made from African wax prints.

Likewise *The Scramble for Africa* (2003) uses dummies dressed in Dutch wax, a fabric that was initially destined for colonial markets in the East Indies, but was introduced to West Africa in the late 1890s. The primary motive was the opening up of new export markets to offset the protectionist trade policies of European nations which prompted the African continent to be carved up into nation states during the final phase of colonialism and initiated the period of direct rule. More recently, Shonibare has transposed African wax prints to scenes of contemporary political events elsewhere. In *Space Walk 2002*, a reconstruction of the Apollo Moon Landings of 1969, the spacemen wear African prints (by then becoming popular with the Black Power movement in America), a device that reveals the existing division between social and technological perspectives of the future. As in *Cha cha cha* and reconstructions of iconic paintings such as Jean-Honoré Fragonard's *The Swing* (2001 [original 1766]) and Thomas Gainsborough's *Mr and Mrs Andrews without their Heads* (1998 [original circa 1750]), which reconstruct paintings of the landed gentry at leisure.

Marcus Amerman (USA), *Art is War Shirt*,
2003. Elk hide with size 13 glass beads.

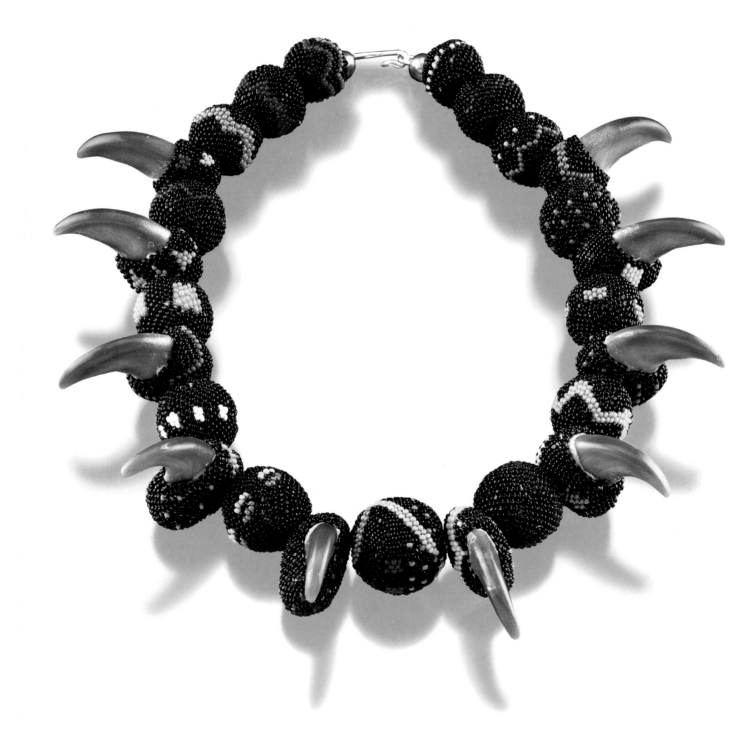

Bear Claw Necklace, 2003. Choctaw beadwork made using size 13 cut beads and peyote stitch. Glass and silver beads were used as trade items from the 16th century onwards.

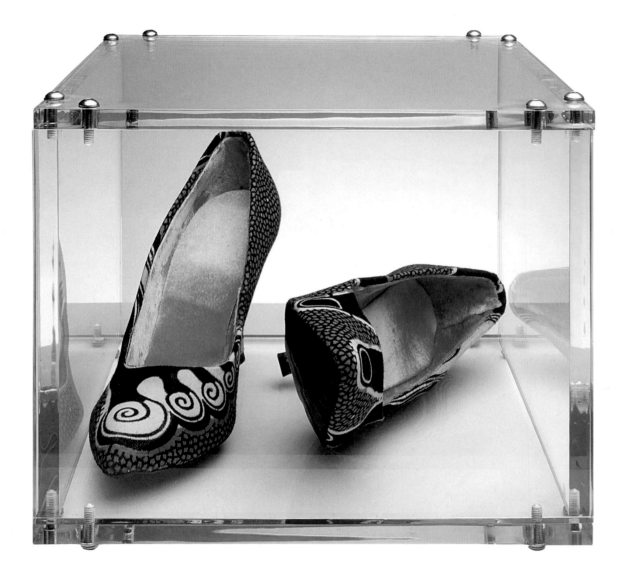

Yinka Shonibare (UK), *Cha cha cha*, 1997.
Stiletto shoes made from Dutch wax-printed
cotton velvet, placed in a riveted perspex
box. Copies of old Dutch wax-resist printed
fabrics, originally developed for sale in West

Africa at the end of the 19th century, were
after factories of African wax cloth.

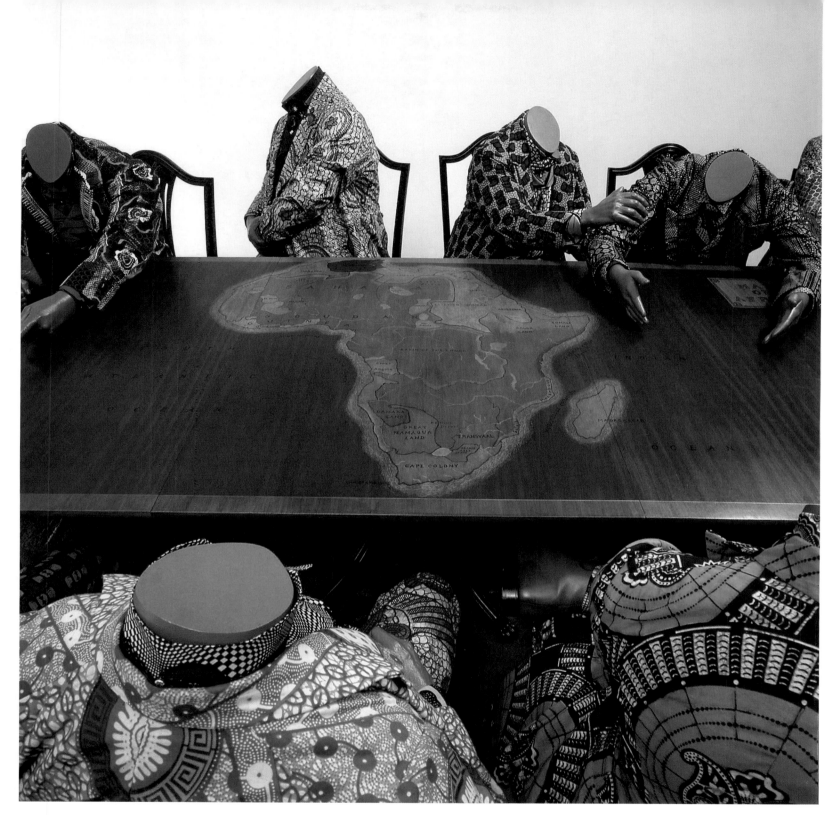

Yinka Shonibare (UK), *Scramble for Africa*, 2003. Fourteen fibre-glass mannekins dressed in African wax prints, commissioned by the Museum for African Art, New York for the exhibition *Looking Both Ways*, courtesy of the artist and the Stephen Friedman Gallery. Developing new export markets for manufactured and traded goods contributed to competing claims for African territory between rival European imperial powers between 1884 and the outbreak of World War One. It was in 1885 that Dutch wax-resist prints, originally made in the Netherlands for sale in the East Indies, began to be traded in West Africa. Soon roller-printed imitations of these fabrics were being specifically designed and manufactured in Manchester for West African markets.

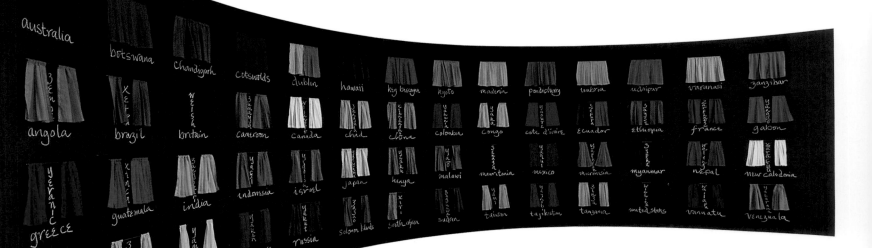

Conceptual Craft

British artists have also investigated the relationship between textiles and cultural identity through dressing up, or through infiltrating vernacular craft traditions. In the late 1990s British artist Grayson Perry worked on a series of embroideries (designed on paper and executed by CAD/CAM or with the aid of an embroiderer) and quilts that suggested how supposedly polite and innocuous decorative traditions deceive us by hiding their malignant and culturally dangerous features. *Mother of all Battles* (1996), in which Perry's cross-dressing alter ego, Claire, poses with a gun in a version of an Eastern European folk costume, was made in the aftermath of the Srebrenica Massacre of 1995, the largest mass murder in Europe since the Second World War, when the Serbian army killed more than 8,000 Bosnian boys and men. In many ways it can be seen as an interpretation of Serbian women's folk dress, in which the conventional use of peonies embroidered in red represents a foundational act of sacrifice: the blood spilt at the semi-mythologized battle conducted against the Ottomans at Kosovo in 1389. In Perry's work the Turkic aspects of Serbian costume are reinterpreted by references to the Palestinian *intifada*: the appliquéd panels show a bombed-out bus at the centre of a Star of David. 'I wanted to make an

Sarindar Dhaliwal, *Curtains for Babel*, mixed media installation, 1996–2006. Dhaliwal was born in the Punjab, raised in England and now works in Toronto.

Grayson Perry (UK), *Mother of All Battles*, 1996 (opposite, above, right), was made in the aftermath of the Srebrenica Massacre in 1995, when 8,000 Bosnian Muslims lost their lives. It portrays Perry's alter ego, Claire, holding an AK-47 while wearing an embroidered dress modelled on Eastern European folk costume. It is one of a series of pieces made by Perry that explore the relationship between vernacular folk art traditions and cultural essentialism through dressing up.

Alicia Framis (Spain), anti-dog collection made from bulletproof Twaron (opposite, below, right and opposite, above, left). Spanish artist Alicia Framis was inspired to make the anti-dog after she was warned not to go walking Marzahn, a suburb of Berlin, for fear that her dark skin would provoke a skinhead attack. Since it was launched at Paris fashion week in 2002, the anti-dog collection has been performed in different venues across Europe.

176   TEXTILES, ART AND CULTURE

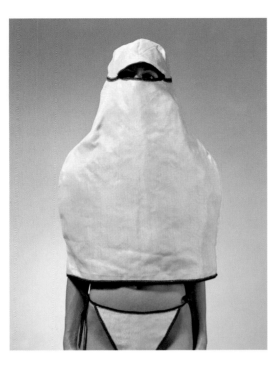

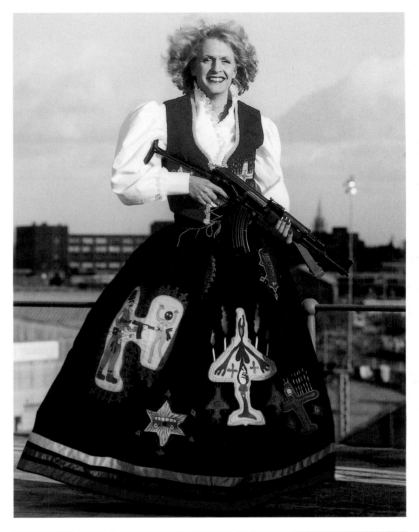

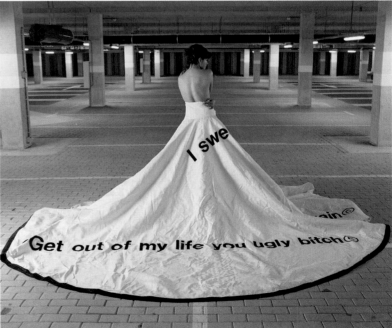

embroidery piece that was as traditional as a vase. Folk costume is an essential element of ethnic identity. Many recent wars and genocides have been about ethnic identity.'

It is one of many of Perry's pieces that conveys textile culture at its most limited, where the meanings of patterns are set, just as the culture it represents has become fixed and unalterable, closed to the inclusion of external elements. In the work of other artists, for instance, British artist Hew Locke's *Menace to Society* (1999), textile crafts such as crochet and embroidery are used as a medium to convey the transgression of conservatism and imperial authority and the imposition of foreign crafts upon the indigenous population. Where craft is used as an instrument of cultural revival it can suggest rather different outcomes however.

Amazwi Abesifazare (Voices of Women) was intended to complement the work of the Truth and Reconciliation Commission by organizing the making and display of a substantial archive of hand-embroidered 'memory cloths' which would record women's individual experiences under apartheid. More than 2,000 cloths have been made by women from the townships and remote rural communities of KwaZulu-Natal, the Eastern Cape, the Free State and the Ganteng

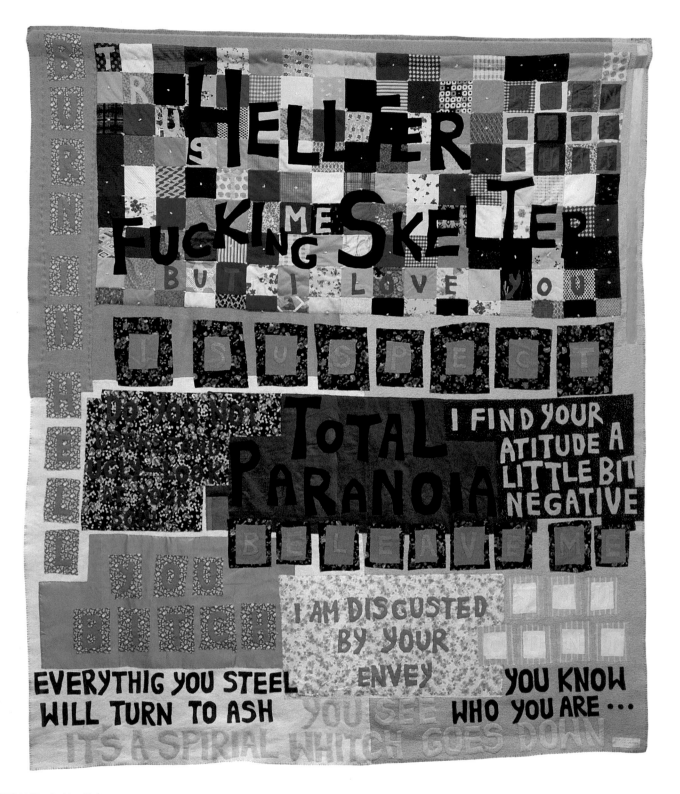

Tracey Emin (UK), *Hellter Fucking Skelter*, 2001.

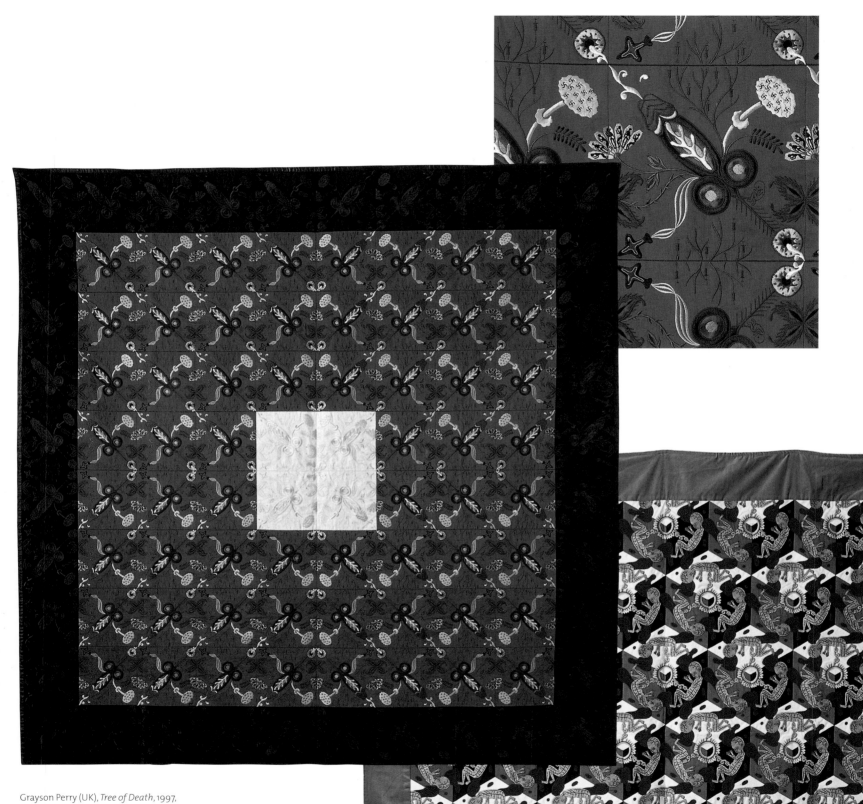

Grayson Perry (UK), *Tree of Death*, 1997, and *Right to Life*, 1997. Cotton and rayon embellished with computer-controlled embroidery.

CONCEPTUAL CRAFT

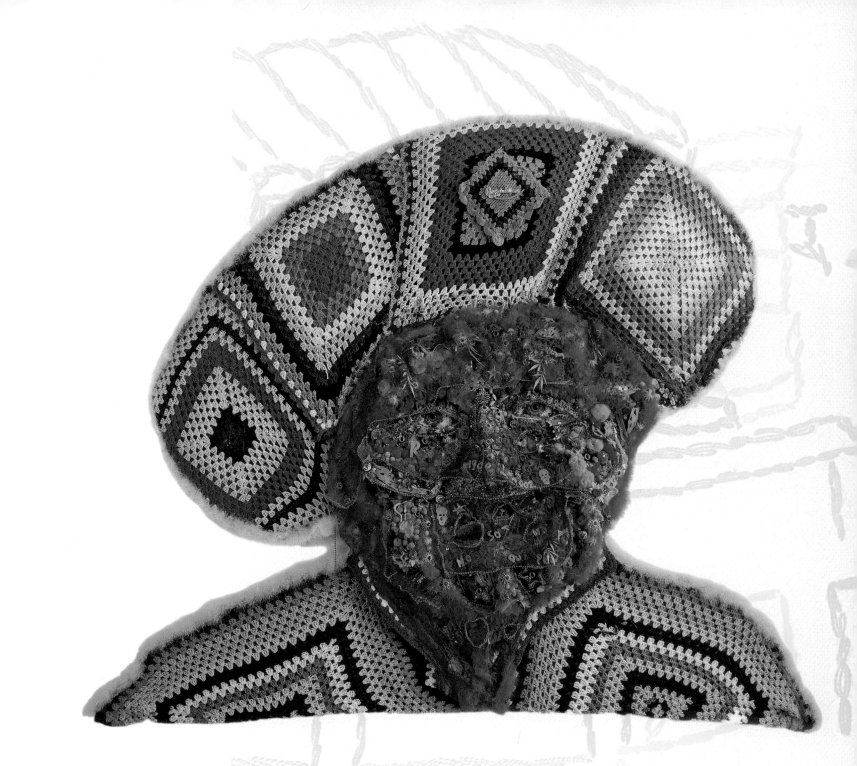

Hew Locke (UK), *RIP*, 2002. Locke was born in Edinburgh and spent his late childhood and early adolescence in British Guiana (modern-day Guyana) where images of British royalty presided on the walls of houses, schools and other administrative buildings. He was expelled from a school in Guyana for drawing a portrait of the Queen on the wall – an experience that has given him a lasting interest in the power of images of authority and the rights that ordinary people can exercise over them. He returned to Britain 20 years ago and now lives in Brixton, London. All the crocheted squares, textiles, beadwork, dolls and other ephemera for his *Menace to Society Series* come from there.

Nomonde Mrwebi (Free State, South Africa), *Amazwi Abesifazane (Voices of Women)*, a project organized by Create Africa South and initiated by Andries Botha. Over 2,000 embroidered 'memory cloths' have been made in KwaZulu-Natal, Eastern Cape, Free State and Gaute ng Provinces.

The day I will never forget in my life.

Growing up comes with a lot of challenges and hardships. It is so hard to grow up without parents. Being brought up by other people usually bears tasteless fruits. Zidwesha, Mlisa and Mthinjane, borrow me your ears so that I can tell you my story concerning the above-mentioned topic.

My parents died when I was five years old. I used to seek shelter from everyone until my uncle took me to stay with him when I was seven. My uncle was rich. He had everything. He had a lot of livestock. I was the darling on the first year that I had arrived. There were

three of us kids at home. There was a boy and another little girl. Things changed as the years went by. Now, before I went to school I would have to fetch water, cook for the dogs and prepare for the other kids to go to school. I would arrive at school at about 9am. There are two unforgettable incidences that happened to me during my stay with my uncle and I will never forget them.

My uncle raped me! The first time he did this was when he told me not to go to school, as he said that I would have to help me in his shop. I was so happy when he told me that I would help him. The entire day was nice. He

fed me with all nice things. We closed the shop at five. He then told me to wait for him in one of the rooms in the back. When he came to me he had a gun. He asked me if I knew that guns kill. I was so scared. He ordered me to take my clothes off. He then raped me to his satisfaction. I had never experienced such pain before. He threatened that if I had told anyone about what had happened he was going to kill me. I was now always lonely. I could hardly play with other children. Teachers were complaining about my change of behavior because I now scared of even the teachers themselves.

When my uncle's wife noticed those changes she ordered me to quit school and concentrate on taking care of the livestock. The second incident was when I had come home at 8am and two sheep had gone missing. He beat and nearly killed me with a sjambok (whip). He told me that I was not going to spend the night inside the house without having found the sheep. I went back to the grazing field even though it was raining and misty. I could hardly see my way. I went to hide myself in an old house that was not occupied anymore. While I was in that house in the middle of the night I heard the

screams of a horse. I also heard footsteps. While I was still shocked and scared I heard a big laugh. Suddenly there were birds flying all over the place and owls crying. I was so scared. I tried to scream but the voice could not come out of my mouth. I cursed my parents for living alone.

I lost my mind for a while. A boy who was herding cattle discovered me. I was dumb for a while. Ghosts had visited me. My leg was broken. The boy rode on his horse and reported to the village what he had seen. A car took me to the hospital and I was given help. The doctor checked me and I told him about what my uncle had done to me.

I spent three months in the hospital. The police went to apprehend my uncle. I was sent to the social workers that took real good care of me. I met other orphans and I forgot about the past. I am still continuing with my subjects now. I will never get out of my mind what happened to me.

Provinces and it is hoped that the total number of cloths will reach 5,000 by 2010. Each cloth is based on the theme of the 'Day I Will Never Forget'. Embroidery and beadwork are used tactically here: they serve as a foil, throwing the stories of violence into relief. But although the medium and the naïve, untutored approach to image-making are affecting, the stories these images tell often describe the more complex side effects of poverty and violence during apartheid rather than stories of direct victimization by Afrikaaners that were being dealt with by the Truth and Reconciliation Commission.

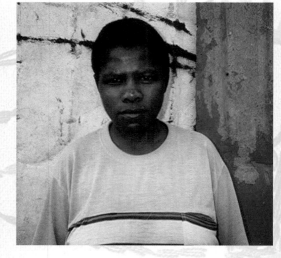

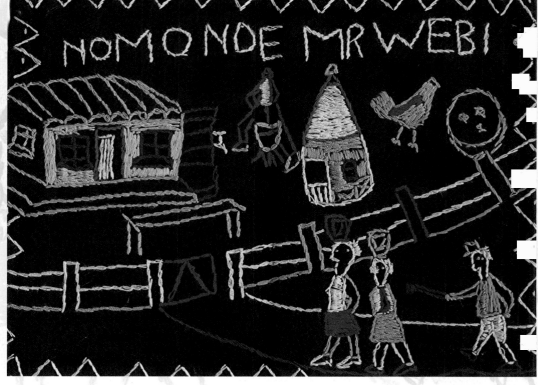

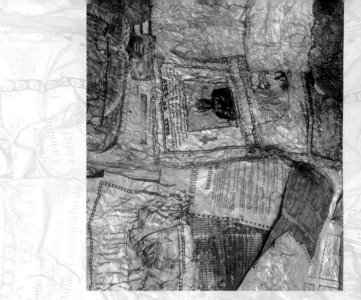

Art and Textile Culture in Nigeria

In other parts of the world the use of textile tradition in cultural revival has involved broadening out the terms of textile culture to embrace different aspects of everyday life. Ghanaian-born artist El Anatsui has represented African cloth in a number of different media such as wood, clay and metal since the early 1970s when he began teaching sculpture at the University of Nigeria on the Nsukka campus. His work may be understood as an exploration of the nature of textile culture. Initially, Anatsui's interest in traditional, or what he calls 'classical African art', began with a study of *adinkra* symbols (pictorial motifs that are stamped on the walls, pots and textiles and logos of the Ashanti people of Ghana). At this point, he was using cloth as a means of researching African iconography, in the hope of finding a distinctive African image language. By the 1980s, however, he had begun to see cloth as a way of conveying something much broader about the transmitted history or culture of a people.

In an interview with the Nigerian art critic Olu Oguibe he said, 'A few years ago we had this go back and pick syndrome in Ghana. In Twi we call it *Sankofa*: "return and retrieve". *Sankofa* syndrome was a reaction to a conscious and forcible attempt to denigrate a people's culture and replace it with an extraneous one.... As in all situations of this kind, it recognised also that there are always elements of an invading culture that stay behind; you cannot obliterate it completely because every culture has its positive aspects. Thus the essence was neither a wholesale return to the past nor a total exclusion of external influence. The thrust was towards inward orientation and selectivity.'

By the 1990s he had begun to connect these aspects of transmitted history to contemporary experience by representing cloth motifs on local found objects, such as the wooden trays used to sell vegetables at the markets, or the rusted sheets of corrugated iron he found on the streets. Such materials helped him to place textile culture in contemporary context. In another interview he explained, 'You know you can memorialise a lot of things in cloth instead of having a statue in bronze or marble, in fact these days cloth is loaded with so much meaning that it is rare to go to a cloth market, for instance, and find a cloth which does not have a name. And the name is not something which has come out of the blue, it's something tied to that place or person or an event that when it is mentioned, you know what is being referred to – it's something in the environment.'

Since the turn of the millennium Anatsui has worked on a series of shimmering, monumental cloths made up from pieces of metal: discarded beer caps and tins of imported European milk, 'Back home we would characterise someone who is given to the pleasures of drinking

El Anatsui, *Wastepaper Bag*, 2003, 'shroud'
made from aluminium lithographic plates
of funerary announcements.

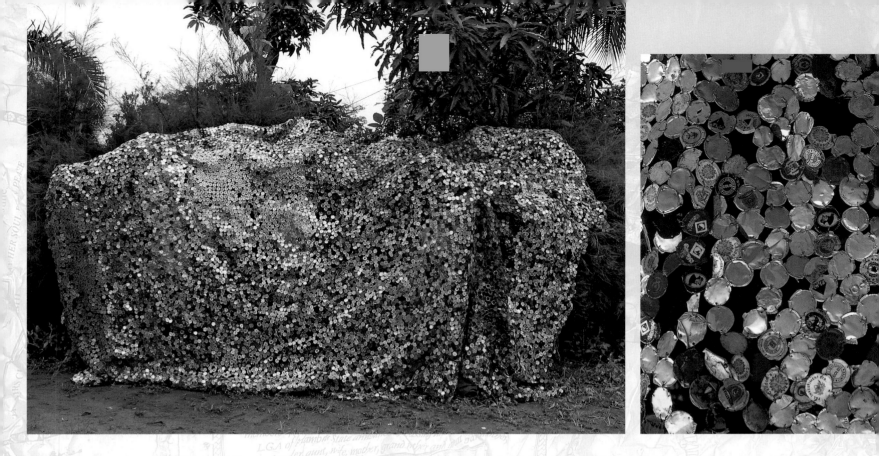

and eating as someone who is "building in the stomach" – the whole piece is...about consumption.... A lot of things which are made in Europe and America and are sent over, arrive in certain kinds of packaging.... Being that you don't have the means to recycle there develop huge piles of milk tins, drink tops and all these things all over the place.'

The gold, red and green metal bottle tops are flattened and sewn into strips that evoke the yellows, reds and greens of *kente* stripwoven royal cloths made by the Akan peoples and in Ghana. 'Art grows out of each particular situation and I believe that artists are better off working with whatever their environment throws up. I think that's what has been happening in Africa for a long time, in fact not only in Africa but the whole world, except that maybe in the West they might have developed these professional materials.... I believe that colour is inherent in everything and it's possible to get colour from around you and that you're better off trying to pick something which relates to your circum-stances and your environment than going to buy a ready made colour.' And one can see why: the transformation of metal into cloth, consump-tion and beer drinking into artistic revival (Ghana was formerly known as the Gold Coast) is both evocative of the past and of the often difficult context of cultural revival in the present.

This approach has inspired a new generation of artists such as Eva Obodo and Dilomprizulike who also make images from local cloth. Lagos-based artist Dilomprizulike creates assemblages from junked clothes and other rubbish that he finds on the streets of Lagos and houses some of his art in a shack he calls 'The Museum for Awkward Things'. His favoured materials are local only in the sense that they have been found locally – they are imported second-hand clothes that have been worn to rags and ribbons on the streets. His is a bleaker vision: he insists that his work has nothing to do with recycling or transformation; the rags in *Waiting for Bus* (2003) portray aspects of life in Lagos as it is.

El Anatsui (Ghana), *Earth Cloth*, 2003.
Liquor bottle cloths, aluminium foil and
copper wire.

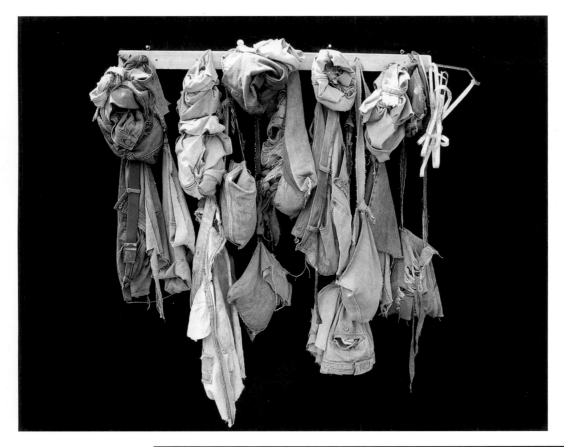

Eva Obodo (Nigeria), *Bricklayer's Wardrobe*, 1997. Made of fabric, wood and a tape measure. The fabric is old, torn jeans collected from friends and tailors' litter bins. The discarded, broken, flexible metal tape measure, the wood and the nails are from a carpenter's shed.

Eva Obodo (Nigeria), *Kata Kata*, 2005. Made of fabric (jute/cotton), metal, enamel paint and a horse whip. The jute sacks, barbed wire, daggers, arrows, crucifix, red enamel paint and horse whip were purchased from a local market, while the stuffing materials were selected from tailors' litter bins.

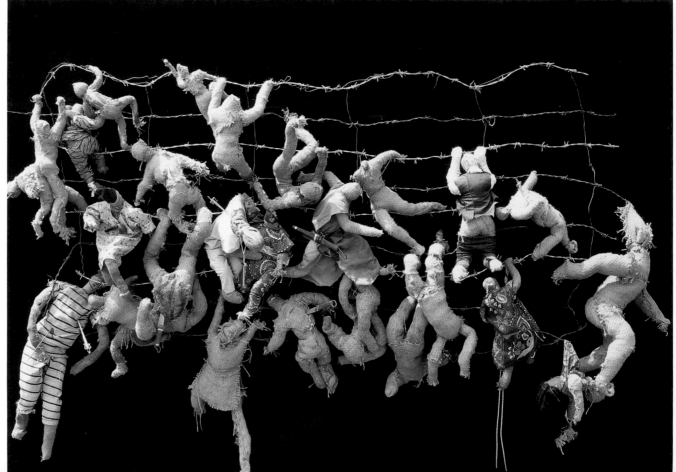

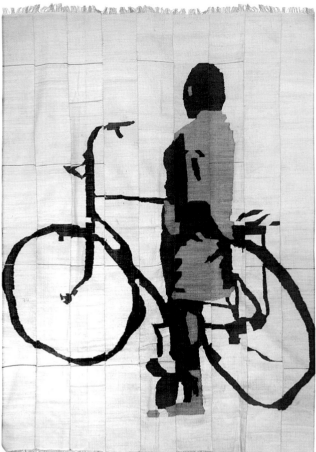

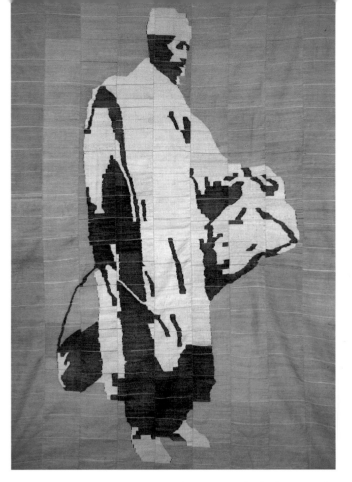

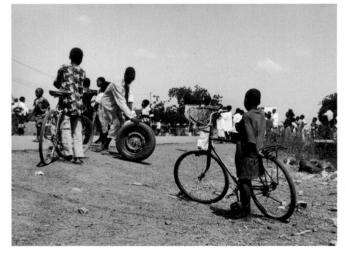

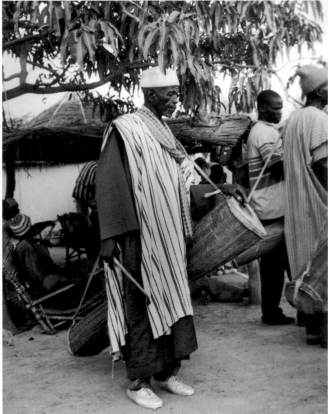

Anthony Labouriaux (France), *Image Tisserands*, 1999–2006, is an ongoing prcject that Labouriaux began working on in 1999 when he first went to live in Koho, a sma`l bush settlement of artisan weavers in Burkina Faso. Having studied the kind of patterns produced by horizontal strip weaving, Labouriaux began to manipulate photographs of weavers digitally.

Textiles and Cultural Exchange in the Pacific Diaspora

The past two decades have shown us that textiles can often tell us more about contemporary culture in the colonial and post-colonial epochs than conventional fine art media. Yet much recent work about cloth has reinforced the view that the contemplation of art is a purely intellectual and aesthetic act: cloth is distanced from clothing; clothing is abstracted from the performer; the act of seeing from the experience of making; and the sensitivity to place and cultural tradition that goes into making textile pieces is constrained by the conventions of display in the gallery system. The relationship between tradition and innovation may have been effectively explored, but perceptions of material culture continue to constrain how complex and heterogeneous art traditions, which may involve not only cloth and other artefacts, but also body art, cooking, food, and performance and dance, are projected on the international contemporary art scene.

The Buddy System (2001–2006) is an interactive installation by New Zealand artist Ani O'Neill that attempts to address some of these issues. Gallery goers are encouraged to sit down in a pleasant and relaxed setting and be taught by a 'buddy' to crochet a flower that will be pinned to the wall to form part of a growing network of flowers. They are then asked to fill out a form identifying their flower and stating the name and address of a family member or a friend that they would like their flower to be sent to after the installation is taken down.

O'Neill's work with 'crafty' materials (a favourite expression) is not shocking like many pieces of conceptual craft from the UK, yet the appearance of innocence is deceptive. Submitting to being taught how to crochet in a gallery setting is a disarming experience – while some people are moved, others are haunted by the sense of triviality – and, since all the 'buddies' have some Polynesian heritage (O'Neill herself was brought up by her Cook Island grandmother), there is also sense of role reversal here. Gallery goers consider the way women from the Pacific Islands were encouraged to take up needlework such as quilting and later crochet in place of their own native arts during the missionary and colonial periods (the form-filling is relevant here), in the belief that a proper pastime might assist in the process of moral redemption. Even O'Neill's approach to image-making has a duality to it, at once acquainted with the contemporary art debates and evocative of the sociable dimension of Pacific ceremonial exchange in which the assembly and distribution of cloth images and food becomes an act of communion and commemoration that makes one think of past and present, of oneself and others.

O'Neill was a member of a performance group called 'The Pacific Sisters' who worked on a diverse range of projects involving cloth and clothing that included fashion styling, designer making, performance and contemporary art, and photography and documentary between the

Contemporary artist Ani O'Neill (New Zealand) has a distinctive approach to working with textiles that comes from being taught to crochet, sew and knit in the company of her Cook Island grandmother. Her way of working shows that there is more to Pacific culture than objects: instead, making textiles becomes an occasion for people from different places to sit down together, converse and reflect upon the nature of the relationship that exists between them.

The Buddy System, 2001–2006, is an interactive installation based on crochet, one of many cottage industries that have been taken up and adapted in the Pacific.

The installation evokes the commemorative dimension of making and presenting textile displays at ceremonial exchanges in the Pacific, which often involves story telling, as well as other ways of enacting the ancestral past – but to a foreign audience and in a contemporary art gallery. In New York, where *The Buddy System* was mounted at Art in General in 2005, visitors were helped to make a crocheted flower by a 'buddy': either O'Neill or her assistant, Megan Ruth Hansen Knarhoi, who also has a Polynesian background. This was then added to a growing vine of flowers on the gallery wall. At the end of the installation the vine was dismantled and the flowers were sent to friend or relation specified by the participant.

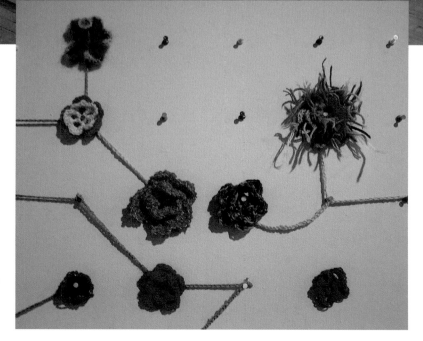

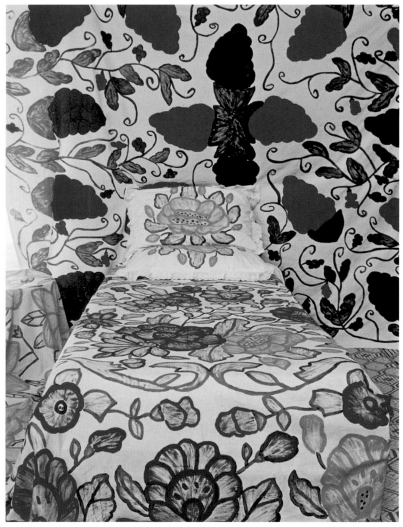

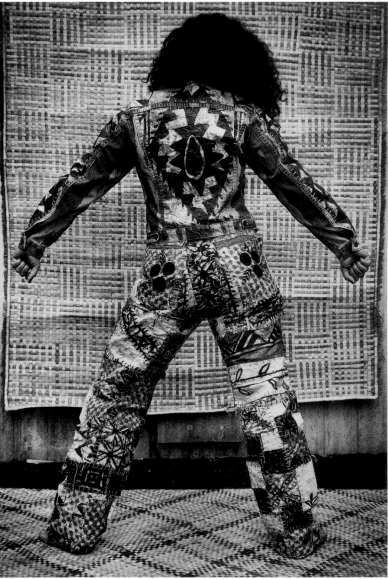

Women's annual tivaevae exhibition, Seventh Day Adventist Churches, Titikaveka, Rarotonga, the Cook Islands, 2003.

Rosanna Raymond (New Zealand/UK), *Gnang Gnear Levi Suit* customized with reclaimed Tongan barkcloth. In the late 1980s, Raymond felt that the representation of Polynesian culture in New Zealand was out of step with what was happening in the Auckland youth scene. Her work as a fashion stylist, performer and designer maker with the co-operative 'The Pacific Sisters' challenged these limitations. The tapa Levis shown here are patched with reclaimed Tongan barkcloth – a traditional exchange valuable. Large quantities of barkcloth and mats are exported from the Kingdom of Tonga and other islands in the Pacific to members of expatriate communities in New Zealand for use at family gatherings. When she hosted *Pasifika*, a showcase of new Pacific fashion design at the Auckland Festival of the Arts, she broke new ground by incorporating aspects of Polynesian performance in the mannequin parade. This approach extends to her work as a stylist. The pose of this model is reminiscent of an iconic photograph of Elvis, but she is also turning away from the camera, subverting the conventions of photographing Polynesian women that date back to cartes de visite from the 1870s onwards.

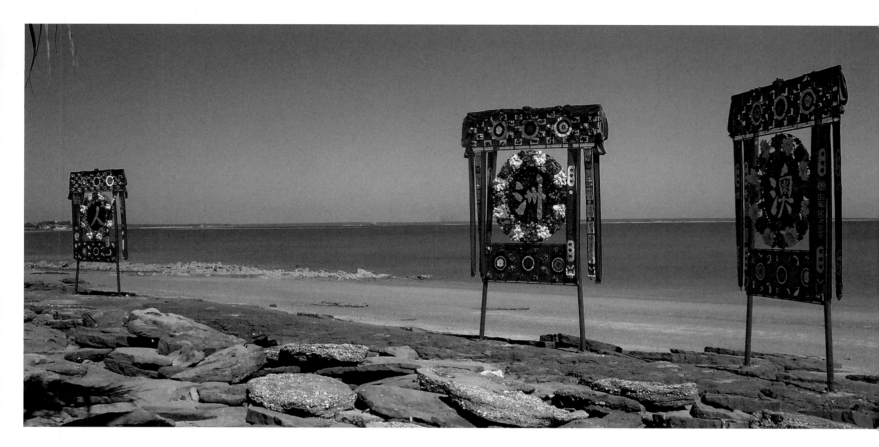

early 1990s and the turn of the century. The venues they chose for their work were deliberately varied – styling magazines, fashion festivals, performances in art galleries, street performances, installations in abandoned housing, street markets and cultural festivals which are such a large part of contemporary Pacific culture. One of their members, Rosanna Raymond, helped to popularize the idea of a distinctive Pacific approach to fashion aesthetics by launching a fashion show 'Pacifica' in Auckland in 1991 which incorporated Pacific textiles and the elements of performance and even clowning that are often a feature of cloth performances in the islands. *Gnang Gnear*, styled by Raymond, conveys this approach well. Here the model adopts an Elvis pose (Elvis was immensely popular among many Pacific Islanders) while wearing a tapa levi suit, patched together from sections of Tongan barkcloth that were put out for recycling after big family gatherings in the suburbs of Auckland.

Global Fashion/Local Tradition – the title of an exhibition mounted in Utrecht in 2005 by Jan Brand and José Teunissen quotes the formula – the opposition between universal modernity and a local cultural tradition in which tradition guides the assimilation of a global universal form is often used to assess innovative work such as Raymond's. Yet it is this static and unitary view of cultural tradition that Raymond is trying to escape from, through recycling barkcloth that has nothing to do with her own mixed Pacific Island and Maori ancestry, and which is furthermore a cloth that is neither culturally unique nor universal in the first place; it is the product of the import and export of ideas and garments during the missionary and colonial periods.

Cold Power T-shirt by Shigeyuki Kihara (another member of The Pacific Sisters) conveys what it must feel like to have one's history denied. Her T-shirt is printed with the instructive cartoon (intended to

Greg Kwok Keung Leong, *The Sojourners*, 2005. Commissioned by the Museum and Art Gallery of the Northern Territory and exhibited on the foreshore outside the museum, where many of the first Chinese migrants to Australia arrived during the 19th century. *The Sojourners* is fashioned in the style of Chinese ceremonial banners and funerary wreaths.

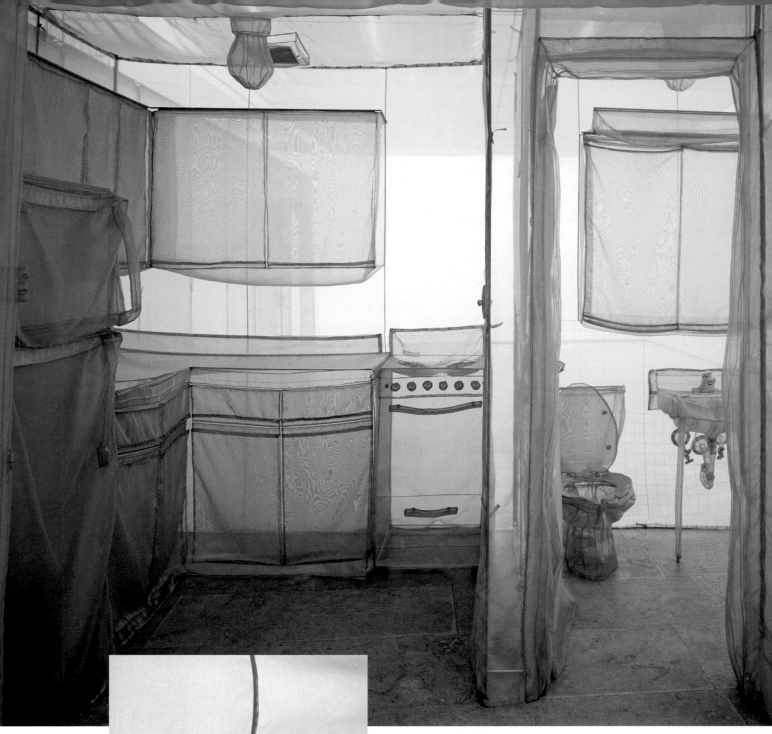

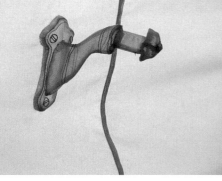

Do-Ho Suh (South Korea) has established an international reputation in recent years for sewing detailed replicas of his home in Seoul from fine silk. *Perfect Home II*, 2003, is an exact replica of the artist's Manhattan apartment sewn from pastel-coloured net curtain material as if it were a garment that could be packed into a suitcase. The hallway is pink while the flat itself is made from pale blue netting. The way the artist has rendered taps, light switches, kitchen units (above) and even the Philips head screws (left) on the doors reveal his attention to detail – what is missing are any of the artist's personal belongings.

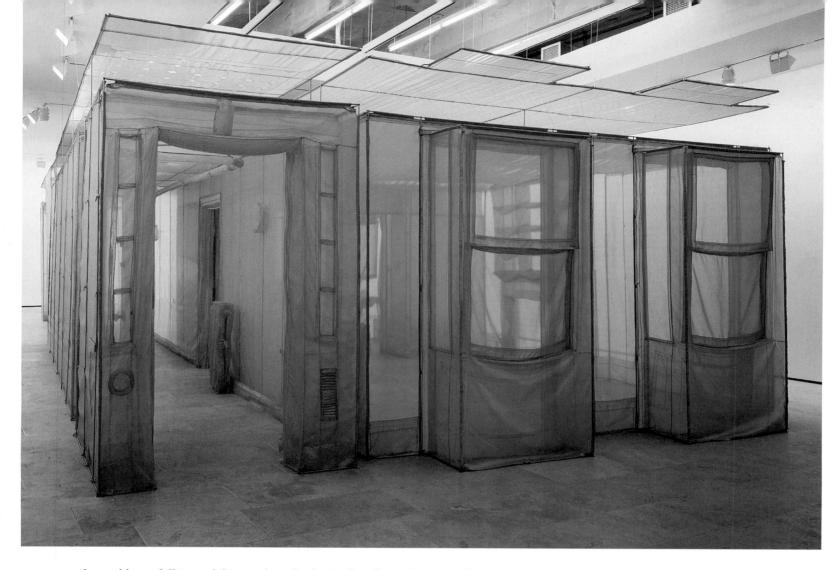

overcome the problem of illiteracy) featured on the back of packets of Cold Power soap. It shows women how to use the product, but women have been hand washing the family laundry the live long day for over a century, just as long as they have been reading the Bible in fact.

If African wax fabrics or Hudson Bay Blankets are redolent of the last phase of colonialism, T-shirts (an item of French underclothing that was issued to the US Army in the Second World War, which are now primarily manufactured in China) have come to stand in many peoples minds for globalization and the relentless extension of American mass consumer culture to the more remote regions of the earth in the second half of the 20th century. In the past twenty years they have become

a standard item of traditional dress across the Pacific, as the photographic project in the remote Asmat region of Irian Jaya by Dutch photographer Roy Villevoye indicates. But what kind of universal form are they? T-shirt graphics have evolved as they have passed out of the American mainstream and crossed over from one section of the population to another, developing from their use in US political and advertising campaigns in the 1960s to the international use of T-shirts for political protest and counter cultural expression such as logo subversion during the 1980s and 1990s.

Designs by T-shirt artists who are descended from Samoan migrants in Auckland draw upon many graphic strands that have

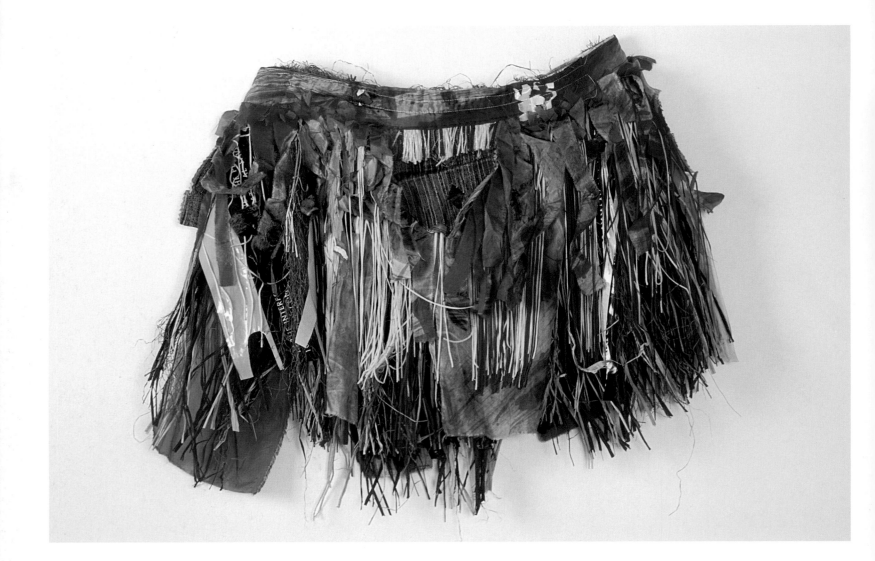

Wendi Choulai (Australia), *105 Skirt*, 1996.
Made of raffia sago palm and girls' plastic
sports' bags, Choulai's grass skirt was
worn at a ceremonial performance at the
third Asia Pacific Triennale. It combines
traditional and introduced materials.

TEXTILES, ART AND CULTURE

Walter van Beirendonck (Belgium),
embroidered redingote for his *Relics from the
Future collection*, Summer 2006. Beirendonck
took inspiration from Captain Cook's
encounter with the Easter islanders. Many
European designers see Pacific Island culture
either in general terms or in the past tense.

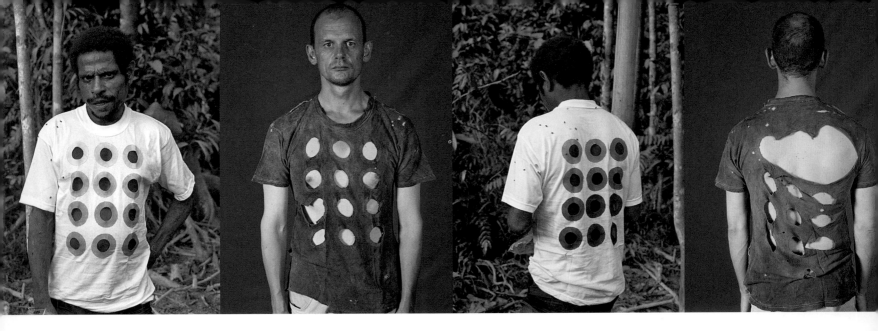

developed through the countercultural use of T-shirts in the United States, such as the use of T-shirts in the rap music scene and the kind of logo subversion that became popular through surf and later the skateboard scenes – two genres that were later taken up by Rez Dog (Mary and Keith DeHaas) to convey the contemporary nature of humour in Native American reservations. By drawing on these elements of T-shirt graphics, the designs accurately convey the complex relation to place and terms of reference experienced by the younger generation of descendants of Samoan migrants in Auckland, whose education may well have involved visits to relatives in the home islands, as well as to relatives living on the West Coast of America and a period of study in Hawaii. Their designs subvert commercial signage of McDonalds, Kentucky Fried Chicken, Coke, Corn Beef, American Express consumer products that entered the cultural traditions of Western Samoa through the use of the islands as a US military base, but which are also a feature of the bland suburbs of South Auckland where they are based.

Visual and verbal analogy is a recurrent theme that is used to probe deeper issues of cultural similarity and difference. American Express becomes Samoan Express, the roadworks sign resembles the earth ovens used by Polynesians to bake pigs for ceremonial occasions. These resemblances are funny because they cut across the Pacific Islanders who typically discuss cultural difference by opposing 'The Way of the Land', i.e., the often idealized simple way of life in the Pacific Islands and 'The Way of Money', the alien consumer culture of the foreign way of life; this convention of speech allows the children of migrants from the Pacific Islands who were initially teased by both Maori and New Zealanders for their provincialism to assert their cosmopolitanism.

The cosmopolitan references and the style of humour, 'turning the negative positive', is at once sophisticated and self-deprecating, an approach that conveys their response to living in the bi-cultural nation of Aotearoa, New Zealand, now formally recognized as the homelands of the Maori. In contrast to the cultural essentialism that was used by the Maori as a rallying point during the 1980s, Samoan T-shirt designers promote an identity that is complex, multifarious and managed – a way of being modern that is not only local, but is also connected to many experiences of modernity. Of course it suits their work, and our sense of textiles in the world, that the T-shirt graphics they work with bring the United States, China and the Pacific together. Was it different in the 19th century? The hybrid, creolized character of many Pacific Island traditions of embroidery and quilting, which were often adopted strategically rather than being imposed by European missionaries, suggests that it was not, though these traditions have only recently attracted attention.

Roy Villevoye (Netherlands), Returning documents: a personal exchange that took place between 1992 and 1997.

'The first time I went to Asmat in Papua, in 1992, I decided to take a few T-shirts with me as presents. They were just ordinary white T-shirts with holes punched through them and a different skin-coloured circle of make-up around each hole.

I was trying to make a tangible painting that would gain new meaning in everyday life. Whoever accepted my T-shirt as a present would complete the work of art by placing the range of skin tones against his own skin when they put the T-shirt on. Excitedly, I took a few photos when the first person donned his present.

After returning home, I started to live with those photos and I kept asking myself who that man was.

Three years later I returned to his village in the rain forest, in the hope of meeting him again. On arrival, I heard that the man, Foyalé Givanep, had died some time previously. Later, when they showed me the remains of the T-shirt I had given him I felt bewildered. So I exchanged it for the shirt I was wearing and took it home with me. Some time after that, I had my photo taken wearing that same T-shirt, as a tribute to that man and also to allay the confusion I felt.

It took two years before I could put the two sets of photographs together.'

Roy Villevoye (Netherlands), *Red Calico*, 1998–2000, photographic project documenting T-shirt customization in the village of Er in Asmat, Papua Province, Indonesia. Asmat sculptors are renowned world wide for their incised carved shields and ancestor boards, many of which are now collectors' pieces. They customize T-shirts by working rents in the surface of the cloth and layering garments on top of each other. They are, from left to right, Matius Serambi, Lambertus Bes and Maria Toyandir, all photographed in 2000.

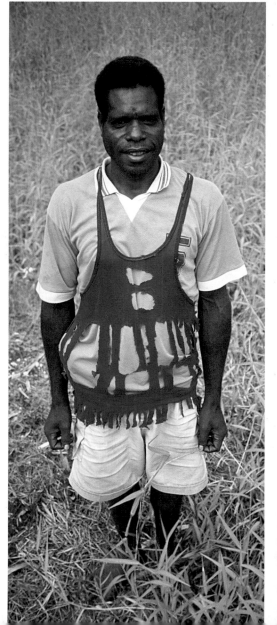
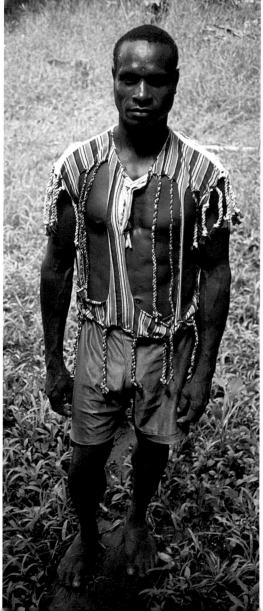
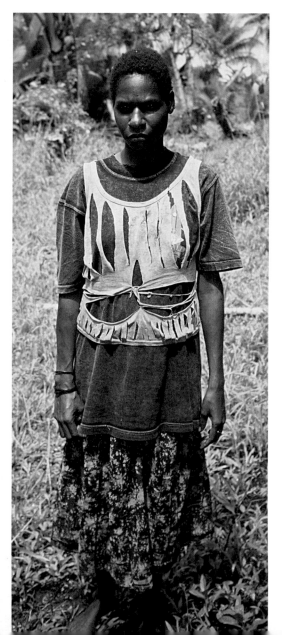

Rez Dog Clothing Company, *Uncivilized*, 2006, and *Does not Assimilate Well into Other Cultures*, 2006.

Mary DeHaas (Fort Peck Assiniboine and Sioux) and Keith DeHaas (Standing Rock Lakota Sioux, USA) founded the Rez Dog Clothing Company in 1996. They began designing T-shirts after attending pow-wow dance festivals in Oklahoma and seeing what they describe as mystic Indian T-shirts.

Rez Dog Clothing plays on the ambiguities of contemporary identity politics to achieve comic effects: self-derogatory in-jokes that are a common to

Indian Reservation humour are offset with its polished cosmopolitanism. The company was recently voted vendor of the year by powwow.com.

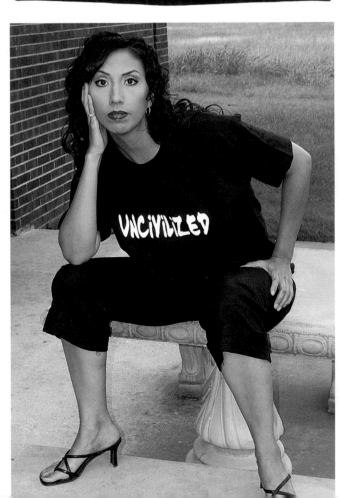

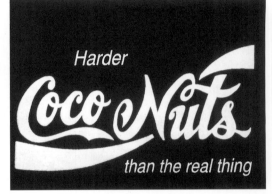

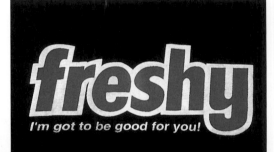

Shigeyuki Kihara (Aotearoa/New Zealand), *Cold Power Cartoon*, 2000, from *Teunca'i-Adorn to Excess Collection* (opposite, above left). Logo Jamming is a marked feature of Urban Pacific Style in Auckland. Typically, it harnesses the power of multi-national brands such as Nike and McDonalds for its subversive effects. Here Kihara, who grew up in Samoa, has harnessed the power of a local brand – Cold Power detergent is used for hand washing throughout the Pacific islands – for comic effect.

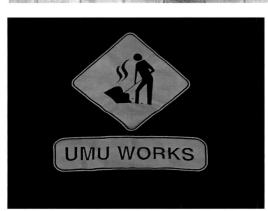

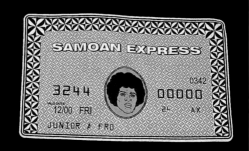

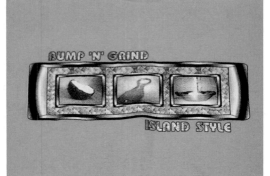

Dean Purcell (New Zealand), *Samoan Express Pacific Gear*, 2000, *Umu Works*, 2001, and *Caution! Coconut Approaching!*, 2000. Modelled by the designer, standing in front of his company logo, under Mangere Bridge in Auckland.

Purcell launched Nektar Clothing in the late 1990s, making analogies that are sparky and pertinent. A local sign showing builders at work is made to resemble an UMU or earth oven, used for baking pigs at ceremonial feasts, by the addition of two wisps of smoke.

Many of Purcell's designs, such as *Bump 'n' Grind* (2001) feature the sort of in jokes and innuendo that offset the deference expected to elders in Samoan culture.

Seliga Setoga (New Zealand), *Freshy – I'm got to be good for you!*, 2000, and *Harder Coco Nuts than the Real Thing*, 2000. Economic migration from the Pacific Islands to Auckland has grown steadily since the 1960s onwards. Initially many of the immigrants were teased for their provincialism by being called Coconuts, or Freshies. Now the offspring of Samoan migrants are getting their own back by designing and making witty T-shirts that turn such comments on their head. Their designs are both localized and cosmopolitan: weaving specific references to Auckland and the relationship between the United States and Samoa, with features of T-shirt design from the surfing, skateboarding and hip-hop scenes in the United States.

Setoga began to design and print his own T-shirts under the label Popo Hardwear at the end of the 1990s. He sold them through his stall at a Polynesian street market in the meat-packing district of South Auckland. As well as localizing logo subversion in a telling manner (Fresh Up, for example, is New Zealand's version of Sunny Delight), Setoga's designs – such as his spoof entry in a dictionary of slang – are semantically complex.

Biographies

Marcus J. Amerman (b. USA, 1959). Amerman is a leading Native American artist whose practice encompasses beadwork, performance and fashion. He comes from a family of beadworkers and became a skilled beadworker himself at the age of 11. His pictorial and satirical beadworks address themes of identity and representation. His work has been featured in seminal exhibitions on contemporary Native American art including: *Who Stole the Tee Pee?*, National Museum of the American Indian, Smithsonian Institution, New York (2000–2001); *Fusing Traditions: Transformations in Glass by Native American Artists*, Museum of Craft and Folk Art, San Francisco (2002) and *Changing Hands: Art Without Reservation II*, the Museum of Arts and Design, New York (2005).

El Anatsui (b. Ghana, 1944). El Anatsui makes sculptures from commonplace objects, creating works that address the contemporary relevance of the rich cultural traditions of the West African coast. He is regarded as one of the leading luminaries of the Nsukka School. He began working in the sculpture department on the Nsukka Campus of the University of Nigeria as a lecturer in 1975 after studying sculpture at the College of Art, University of Science and Technology in Kumasi, Ghana. His work has been exhibited internationally at seminal exhibitions such as *Encounters with the Contemporary*, National Museum of African Art, Smithsonian Institution, Washington DC. (2001) and *Africa Remix*, Hayward Gallery, London (2005). He is represented by the October Gallery in London.

Joel Andrianomearisoa (b. Madagascar, 1977). Andrianomearisoa entered the Fashion Academy of Antananarivo at the age of 12. His fashion designs were first presented in 1995. He has been studying architecture at Paris University since 1998. In 2000 he staged performances at the Centre Georges Pompidou and the Musée d'Art Moderne de la Ville de Paris. He lives and works in Madagascar and Paris, and designs costumes and scenery for theatre, film and television. For his fashion collections, Andrianomearisoa experiments with materials such as wood, metal, stone and plastics, usually associated with sculpture rather than fashion design. He applies the concept of 'archi-couture', using geometrical and radical forms, and creates object-garments that are mostly black. He also uses unusual and exclusive woven materials.

Manish Arora (b. India, 1972). Described as the John Galliano of India, Arora's designs are street savvy and kitsch. While many Indian fashion designers re-create Mughal-style clothing for formal functions such as weddings, Arora has broken free, creating finely crafted contemporary clothes for an international market. His designs exploit the full potential of the rich textile craft traditions of New Delhi. He launched his Manish Arora label in 1997 and a second label Fish Fry in 2001. He was part of the spectacular show on kitsch at the Habitat Centre in New Delhi in 2001. Since September 2005 he has shown his collections at London Fashion Week.

Martín Ruiz de Azúa (b. Spain, 1965). An internationally acclaimed conceptual and experimental designer, his visionary designs look at the way people relate to each other and to the material and physical environment. His work has been exhibited at Vitra and at the Museum of Modern Art, New York. His collaborative work with Gerard Moliné, with whom he formed the design consultancy Azuamoline in 2002, was exhibited in a show entitled *Neo Rural* at the Ego Gallery in Barcelona.

Hildur Bjarnadóttir (b. Iceland, 1969). Bjarnadóttir studied fine arts at the Icelandic School of Arts and Crafts and received her MFA at the Pratt Institute in New York. She learnt to crochet, sew and knit when she was four years old. Her fibre art embraces decorative art, craft and conceptual approaches.

Tord Boontje (b. Netherlands, 1968). Boontje studied industrial design at the Design Academy of Eindhoven (1986–1991) before studying for an MA at the Royal College of Art, London. Studio Tord Boontje was founded in 1996 and its designs for Swarovski, Habitat and Moroso and Kvadrat have spearheaded the re-emergence of a contemporary trend of decoration in industrial design. The current Studio Tord Boontje was set up in Bourg-Argental, France, in 2006.

Bouroullec Brothers (Ronan, b. France, 1971 and Erwan, b. France, 1976). Ronan studied at the Ecole Nationale des Arts Décoratifs in Paris and Erwan at the Ecole Nationale des Beaux Arts of Cergy Pointoise. Their studio is in St Denis, in the suburbs of Paris. Their work, which includes jewelry, office furniture systems and conceptual pieces of architectural scale, is distinguished by the inventive use of form and materials. Many of their projects are composed of repeating elements that can be stacked to occupy large volumes. Their *Polystyrene House* is a conceptual design for housing assembled from foam sections that slot together; their *Floating House* project for an island on the Seine consists of an elongated timber trellis mounted on a barge; Algues designed for Vitra in 2004 is comprised of individual strands of plastic algae that can be assembled together to form a room divider. Their many commissions have included work for Issey Miyake, Cappellini and Habitat. Their designs have been exhibited widely and their solo exhibitions include *Ronan and Erwan Bouroullec* at the London Design Museum in 2002.

Bob Boyer (Canada, 1948–2004). Metis artist Boyer was best known for his *Blanket Statements*, politically charged paintings on blankets that use art as a prism to examine Native American traditions in a post-colonial context. His work draws upon geometric forms found in traditional Native American Plains beadwork and hide painting and comments wittily upon the modernist trend of primary mark marking in American Abstract Expressionism and Colour Field Painting. In 1984, he produced a series of blanket works featured in *Horses Fly Too* at the Mackenzie Art Gallery, Saskatchewan, Canada. Solo exhibitions include *Bob Boyer: A Blanket Statement*, Museum of Anthropology at the University of British Columbia (1988) and *Shades of Difference: The Art of Bob Boyer*, Art Gallery of Alberta (formerly the Edmonton Art Gallery) in 1991.

Michael Brennand-Wood (b. UK, 1952). Brennand-Wood studied at Bolton College of Art and subsequently at Manchester Polytechnic and Birmingham Polytechnic. During the 1980s his brightly hued textile constructions established his reputation as a textile artist of international standing and a major advocate of contemporary craft. Since 2000 he has devoted his attention to floral designs and arrangements that probe the nature of perception. He is currently a research fellow at the University of Ulster.

Wendi Choulai (Papua New Guinea, 1954–2001). A textile designer and performance artist, Choulai studied textiles at the National Arts School Papua New Guinea before moving to Melbourne, Australia, where she studied for an MA in printmaking at RMIT University. Her work was featured at the Asia Pacific Triennale in 1996.

Conserve India. A New Delhi-based NGO that tackles issues of waste management and recycling. It makes bags by heat-pressing used polythene bags through rollers and stitching the panels together. The organization was founded by Anita and Shalabh Aluja in 2003.

Crawford Brewin (UK) Will Crawford and Peter Brewin graduated from the London Royal College of Art's industrial design engineering course in 2005. They invented a building in a bag intended for use by refugees and humanitarian organizations who have to live in tents for months or even years in the wake of a humanitarian disaster. The design has received nine awards including the Saatchi and Saatchi award for World Changing Ideas. In 2005 they founded Concrete Canvas in order to commercialize their invention; in 2006 they received funding from the Department of Trade and Industry and private sponsors to develop pre-production prototypes to be used in the field in 2007.

Sarindar Dhaliwal (b. Punjab, 1953). Dhaliwal was born in Punjab, India, and raised in England. She currently lives and works in Toronto, Ontario.

Eleksen Group Plc (UK). Eleksen are pioneers of conductive fabric-sensing and switching applications. The company researches, develops and licenses soft-sensing and switches technology and product solutions, enabling innovative product development. Their core technology, ElekTex, is an electro-conductive fabric touch pad.

Eley Kishimoto (Japan/UK). (Mark Eley, b. UK, 1968 and Wakako Kishimoto, b. Japan, 1965). Eley studied weaving at Brighton Polytechnic. Kishimoto received a BA and MA in fashion and print at Central Saint Martins College of Art and Design, London. They have developed an international fashion label on the strength of their distinctive graphic screen-printed fabrics produced in their London studio next to Brixton prison. Their approach to pattern making is economical, witty and distinctive. They began working together in 1992, initially working for the textile design consultants Hodge and Sellers and Joe Casley Hayford before establishing their own label in 1996. In 2003 the Victoria and Albert Museum in London staged a retrospective show of their work in *Fashion in Motion*.

Yoel Fink (b. Israel, 1966). Fink is a principal investigator in the Research Laboratory of Electronics (RLE) at the Massachusetts Institute of Technology (MIT). He attended the Technion (Israel Institute of Technology) and received his BSc in Chemical Engineering in 1994, followed by a BA in Physics in 1995. In 2000, he received his PhD in Materials Science from MIT and joined the MIT faculty as Assistant Professor. In 2004, he was promoted to Thomas B. King Associate Professor of Materials Science. Fink's doctoral research examined the theory and synthesis of block copolymer self-assembled photonic band gap materials, as well as the theory and synthesis of dielectric, omnidirectional reflectors (the 'perfect mirror'). In 1998 he developed a way of manufacturing dielectric mirrors in the form of hair-like fibres. In 1999, MIT's Technology Review named him one of the top 100 young innovators under the age of 35. In 2004, Fink won the National Academy of Sciences Award for Initiatives in Research for his pioneering contributions and ingenuity in the creative design and development of photonic materials and devices.

Forsythe MacAllen (Canada). Stephanie Forsythe and Todd MacAllen studied architecture at Dalhousie University in Halifax, Nova Scotia. They formed their architectural partnership in 1998 and later extended their practice to include product design. Molo Design was founded in 2003 and their design, *Softwall*, received the Index Award in 2005.

Freitag Lab AG Zurich (Switzerland). Markus and Daniel Freitag initially started making messenger bags in their flat in 1993. They were living next to the main transit route linking Germany and Italy and thought of a use for truck tarpaulins. The brothers now manufacture a range of bags and suitcases that are marketed internationally, as well as being sold from their flagship stores, one of which is fashioned from used containers.

Shelly Goldsmith (UK). Goldsmith studied woven textiles at West Surrey College of Art and Design, and received a distinction for her MA in tapestry from the Royal College of Art in London. She was awarded the Jerwood Applied Arts Prize for textiles in 2002. A skilled tapestry artist, Goldsmith also uses other techniques such as installation and heat-transfer printing to convey her ideas. Aspects of the lifecycle and the nature of cultural transmission are recurrent themes of her work. She teaches textile art at Winchester School of Art.

Grado Zero Espace (Italy). A company that specializes in transferring technological material and know-how from the research sphere to the industrial domain. It adapts technologies developed by the European Space Agency and the medical and building industries for new everyday uses. The company acts as a go-between among many industrial branches and research fields – such as universities, test labs, the European Space Agency and single researchers and inventors. They have developed a new system of spinning and weaving the bast of stinging nettles (*Urtica Dioica*), a common plant already used in the past as an alternative to cotton. Another development is 'Oricalco', a self-ironing shirt woven from a shape memory alloy called Nitinol which was selected by *Time Magazine* as one of the best inventions in 2001. In 2003 they developed UV protective suits for children affected by Xeroderma Pigmentosum.

Julie Graves (b. UK 1959). Graves studied textiles at Goldsmiths, University of London, and is now the digital archivist for the Constance Howard Resource and Research Centre in Textiles.

Thomas Heatherwick (b. UK, 1970). Heatherwick trained as a designer at Manchester Metropolitan University and at the Royal College of Art, London. He is a Royal Designer for Industry, a Senior Fellow of the Royal College of Art and was awarded an honorary doctorate by Sheffield Hallam University. His practice embraces product design and architecture. Many of his designs have moving parts and show an appreciation for organic form. *Zip Bag*, for example, is an apparently plain leather handbag, which when unzipped doubles in size and reveals a spiral of colour. It went into production in 2003 and was launched at London's Design Museum, becoming a bestseller for Longchamp. Heatherwick Studio was later asked to design Longchamp's first contemporary flagship store, La Maison Unique in SoHo, New York. Heatherwick Studio's Rolling Bridge, designed for an offshoot of the Grand Union Canal in New York, curls back on itself to create a sculptural form.

Linda Hutchins (b. USA, 1957). Hutchins studied computer engineering at the University of Michigan and worked as a software programmer for Intel during the early 1980s before taking a degree in drawing at the Pacific Northwest College of Art in Portland, Oregon. Many of her works develop the understanding of the nature of pattern, repetition and human error that she developed as a computer programmer. Cogitations about the role of cloth in culture are also a recurrent theme of her work. Between 1996 and 2003 she worked on a series of weavings made from plastic barricade tape. In 2004 her experiments with the patterns derived from repeatedly hand typing phrases on paper or cloth were exhibited in the solo exhibition, *Linda Hutchins: Reiterations* at the Art Gym Gallery 2, Marylhurst, University in Oregon. More recently, she has experimented with creating meditative and repetitive line drawings of the sinuous movement of cloth or water.

Sundaresan Jayaraman (b. India, 1954). Jayaraman is a Professor of Textile and Fibre Engineering at the Georgia Technology Institute in Atlanta, Georgia. He received his

PhD from North Carolina State University in 1984 and MTech and BTech degrees from the University of Madras, India, in 1978 and 1976, respectively. In September 1994, he was elected a Fellow of the Textile Institute (UK). In 1996, in response to an appeal by the US Navy, he began work on the development of a smart shirt. Dubbed 'the Georgia Tech Wearable Motherboard', his design was regarded as a major innovation and was judged one of the most important innovations of the year by *Time Magazine* in 2001.

Hella Jongerius (b. Netherlands, 1963). Jongerius studied at the Academy for Industrial Design in Eindhoven and launched her own company, Jongerius Lab, in 2000. Her design practice embraces furniture, tableware, textiles and product design. She is interested in the expressive potential of materials and manufacturing technologies and in the nature of decorative traditions. She rarely creates new forms, but seeks to find ways of using existing forms and techniques to create something new. She has recently worked for Maharam and Royal Tichelaar Makkum. Her work has been internationally exhibited and in 2005 she was asked to select pieces from the Cooper-Hewitt National Design Museum at the Smithsonian Institution, New York, for a solo show.

Sheila Kennedy (b. USA, 1957). Kennedy received an MA in Architecture at Harvard University Graduate School of Design. In 1988 she founded Kennedy + Violich Architecture in conjunction with Frano Violich. Their architectural practice explores the relationship between new material technologies and emerging needs. MATX, the material research wing of their architectural practice, seeks to develop new design solutions by applying the development of energy-efficient digital technologies to architecture. Kennedy's recent projects have encouraged people to rethink the potential uses of light-emitting textiles and photovoltaics. In 2005 Kennedy led the *Portable Light Project* at the University of Michigan which led to the development of a series of prototypes for portable cloth lights that could be of use to the nomadic communities of the Sierra Madre. In August 2006 the practice developed a *Soft House* for the Vitra design museum which uses energy harvesting and light-emitting textiles as moveable textile screens, room enclosures, curtains and blankets.

Shigeyuki Kihara (b. Samoa, 1975). Kihara explores themes of identity, representation and cross-cultural dynamics. Her work encompasses performance, print, contemporary art and fashion styling. Kihara is of both Samoan and Japanese descent. She was born in Samoa and moved to Auckland at

the age of 16. She trained in fashion design at the Massey Institute of Technology (now Massey University) in Wellington. Five years later a series of her T-shirts that parodied well-known corporate logos entitled *Teunoa'i – Adorn to Excess* was added to the collection of the Te Papa Tongarewa, Museum of New Zealand. Her recent series of photographs exhibited at the Sherman Galleries in Sydney, *Fa'fafine: In a Manner of a Woman* (2005), exploit the conventions of 19th-century portrait photography. Kihara uses her body to reconstruct images in an ethnographic style, portraying both a male and female subject. These works convey constructed notions of gender and its cultural embodiment, asserting Kihara's own identity and status as a Samoan and as a *fa'fafine*. In 2003 Kihara was the Creative New Zealand Emerging Pacific Artist; her work can be found in the collections of Waikato Museum of Art and History, Hamilton, Gus Fisher Gallery of University of Auckland, and in Te Papa Tongarewa, Museum of New Zealand.

Anthony Labouriaux (b. France, 1974). Labouriaux studied product and graphic design at the Ecole Supérieure des Arts Décoratifs de Reims. Since 1999 he has made repeated trips to Burkina Faso where he has undertaken a number of collaborative research projects with a weaving community close to Boromo. In 2004 Labouriaux's designs were featured in *Design Made in Africa*, the first major exhibition of African design in the UK which was shown at the Brunei Gallery, School of Oriental and African Studies, London.

Andreas Lendlein (b. Germany, 1970). Lendlein trained in textile chemistry and macromolecular chemistry and, in 1997, while working at MIT, was the first to develop a biodegradable shape-memory polymer that responds to body temperature. Lendlein returned to Germany in 1998 and co-founded mNemoscience, in Aachen, to commercialize his invention. mNemoscience has now received backing to develop its intelligent suture for commercial production. Since 2004 Lendlein has been professor at the department of medicine, University of Aachen, specializing in the development of medical textiles; he is also a director of the GKSS Research Centre and professor at the University of Potsdam.

Greg Kwok Keung Leong (b. Hong Kong, 1946). Leong studied in Hong Kong before studying fine art at the University of Tasmania, where he is now a lecturer. His working practice encompasses performance, costume making and installation art and addresses themes of identity and displacement. His works have been exhibited widely in Australia.

Hew Locke (b. UK, 1959). Locke spent his childhood and adolescence in Guyana and returned to the UK in the mid-1980s. He studied fine art at Falmouth and at the Royal College of Art, London. Much of his work explores the tensions between Western and non-Western imagery and the power of popular imagery. He is best known for his images of the British royal family which he renders from trimmings and crochet ephemera that he gathers on the streets of Brixton in London, where his studio is located. Locke has had solo shows at the Chisenhale Gallery, London, and at the Walsall Gallery. His work also featured in *Boys Who Sew* at the Crafts Council. He was awarded the prestigious Paul Hamlyn Award in 2000.

David Lussey (b. UK, 1945). Lussey is the inventor of Quantum Tunnelling Composite (QTC), a new class of electrically conductive substance that is extremely sensitive to pressure. Lussey, a former engineer in the Royal Air Force, discovered QTC by accident while attempting to manufacture an adhesive that could conduct electricity. QTC is a material made from particles of a metal (nickel) embedded in a polymer. Its resistance changes dramatically when it is compressed. Uncompressed, it is an almost perfect electrical insulator. When a force is applied, it conducts as well as a metal. His company Peratech Ltd was established in 1996 and the company has received significant venture funding to assist in the development and marketing of QTCs. It has won several prestigious industry awards including the Saatchi and Saatchi Innovation in Communication Award and the Tomorrow's World Industry Award.

Rachael Matthews (b. UK, 1974). An artist-knitter, Matthews creates work in response to rites of passage and storytelling. Cast Off, her London-based knitting club, was established in 2000. The club aims to provide an alternative to the usual and often alienating networks in the world of handicrafts by arranging fun and adventurous knitting meetings and workshops in a range of unusual public settings.

William McDonough (b. Japan, 1951). An American architect and author, McDonough is widely regarded as one of the leading protagonists of sustainable architecture and design in the USA. In conjunction with the German industrial chemist and environmental campaigner Dr Michael Braungart, he founded MBDC in 1995 to promote and shape what he calls the 'Next Industrial Revolution' through the introduction of a new paradigm of sustainable design. Their dictum is that both the materials being used in manufacture as well as the end product should not be merely recyclable, but should be defined as a biological or technical nutrient. Their design consultancy focuses as much upon the materials and processes involved in the manufacture and recycling of products as upon the design of objects per se. They have developed a certification scheme that involves a rigorous process of identifying and assessing materials according to their impact on environmental and human health. McDonough is the author of numerous publications on sustainable design and has documented several case studies where his principles have been applied.

Eva Obodo (b. Nigeria, 1963). Obodo graduated in 1992 from the department of fine and applied arts, University of Nigeria, where he subsequently finished his MFA in soft sculpture. Between 1995 and 1996 he was a guest artist at Afrika Studio, Nsukka. His work has been exhibited locally and internationally since 1990, in joint and solo shows. He has also featured in several group exhibitions including *Prints from Nsukka*, Goethe-Institut, Lagos and Berlin (1990). He was shortlisted and exhibited at the Osaka Triennale (2001). He also participated in the 5th Biennale de l'Art Africain Contemporain, Dak'Art (2002). Since 1996, Obodo has been a senior lecturer in sculpture and drawing in the fine art department, Benue State Polytechnic, Ugbokolo.

Ani O'Neill (b. New Zealand, 1971). O'Neill graduated in 1994 with a BFA in sculpture from Elam School of Fine Arts, Auckland University. She lives and works in Rarotonga, Cook Islands and Auckland, Aotearoa/New Zealand. O'Neill makes objects and stages installations and performances that are about the approach to handicraft work that she learnt from her Cook Island grandmother. The techniques she works with include traditional costume making for celebrations as well as Tivaevae (derived from appliqué and quilt making), embroidery, sewing and crochet – crafts which were originally introduced by missionary wives to the Pacific, but which were subsequently transformed by the women from the Cook Islands and elsewhere. Because of their culturally hybrid character, most of these textiles have conventionally been overlooked by ethnographic museums. O'Neill's work is also implicitly critical of the object fixation of Western museums and she seeks to convey the social aspects of the Pacific way of making textiles through video, site-specific and interactive installations and workshops as well as

performance and installations. A former member of 'the Pacific Sisters' collective, O'Neill's work has recently been shown at Art in General, New York and at *Pasifika Styles* at the Museum of Archaeology and Anthropology, Cambridge.

Lucy Orta (b. UK, 1966). Orta studied fashion and textiles at Nottingham Polytechnic in the mid-1980s and was a fashion stylist before embarking on a career as an artist specializing in sculptural clothing and public performance. She established Studio Orta in 1991, in conjunction with the artist George Orta. Her tent-like architectural garments entitled *Refuge Wear* attracted attention in the 1990s. These were followed by larger clothing sculptures, *Collective Wear*, which were used to stage demonstrations and performances. Her ongoing project *Nexus Architecture* has been staged at site-specific performances at the Venice Biennale (1995) and the Johannesburg Biennale (1997). A former lecturer at the University of Eindhoven, she has been Professor of Fashion at the London College of Fashion since 2002.

Grayson Perry (b. UK, 1960). Perry studied fine art at Portsmouth Polytechnic. He is a postmodern artist whose work comments upon the latent aspects of decorative arts traditions such as ceramics and embroidery. He won the Turner Prize in 2003.

Rosanna Raymond (b. New Zealand, 1972). Raymond currently lives, writes and performs in London. A former member of 'the Pacific Sisters' collective in Auckland, she helped to establish the *Pasifika Styles* show at the Pasifika Festival in Auckland in the late 1990s. Since moving to London, she has been a producer and commentator on contemporary urban Pacific island culture, fusing traditional practices with modern innovations and techniques. In 2006 she was made the Leverhulme artist-in-residence at the Museum of Archaeology and Anthropology, Cambridge, where she co-curated the *Pasifika Styles* exhibition.

Rez Dog Clothing. Mary DeHaas (Sioux/Fort Peck Assiniboine) and Keith DeHaas (Lakota Sioux/Standing Rock) founded Rez Dog Clothing Company in 1996; it is now one of the most visible Native American-owned and operated business in North America. They started designing T-shirt graphics alive with inside jokes and reservation slang and were recently voted 'Pow-wow Vendor of the Year' by powwows.com.

Freddie Robins (b. UK, 1965). Robins tutors in constructed textiles, mixed media in the department of textiles at the Royal College of Art, London. Robins studied knitted textiles at Middlesex Polytechnic and the Royal College of Art, London, graduating in 1989. She established Tait & Style, a design company specializing in embroidered, knitted and felted fabrics, with fellow Royal College of Art graduate, Ingrid Tait, designing fashion and furnishing accessory collections and marketing them worldwide. In 1997 she changed her practice and began concentrating on producing conceptually led knitted textile pieces. In 2005 she co-curated *Knit 2 Together: Concepts in Knitting* for the Crafts Council and *Ceremony* at the Pump House Gallery, Battersea Park, London. She has exhibited extensively within the UK, as well as in Germany, Sweden, the Netherlands, Denmark, Austria and Bangladesh.

Galya Rosenfeld (b. Israel, 1977). Rosenfeld studied jewelry, clothing and product design at the Bezalel Academy of Art and Design in Jerusalem before continuing her studies at the Ecole Nationale Supérieure des Arts Décoratifs in Paris. She established her studio in San Francisco in 2001 and was made professor at the California College of the Arts in San Francisco in 2005. Many of her designs are composed of modular elements of fabric which interlock together. Her work has been exhibited internationally.

Jonathan Saunders (b. UK, 1979). Saunders graduated from Glasgow School of Art in 1999 with a BA in Printed Textiles and subsequently graduated from Central Saint Martins College of Art and Design in London in 2002 with an MA with distinction in Printed Textiles. He uses traditional silk-screening techniques to develop specific fabrics for his collections. Saunders coordinates designing his own label alongside consulting for some of the largest fashion houses in Europe. In September 2005 he presented his fifth show at London Fashion Week.

Yinka Shonibare (b. UK, 1962). Shonibare studied at Byam Shaw School of Art and at Goldsmiths College, London, and participated in seminal exhibitions such as *Sensation* at the Royal Academy of Arts, London (1997). In 2004 he was nominated for the Turner Prize in 2005 and he was awarded an MBE. Shonibare selects works from the Cooper-Hewitt National Design Museum at the Smithsonian Institution, New York. Other exhibitions include *Looking Both Ways: Art of the Contemporary African Diaspora*, Museum for African Art, New York (2003), *Double Dutch*, Boijmans van Beuningen Museum,

Rotterdam, Netherlands, touring to Kunsthalle Vienna, Austria (2004), *Africa Remix*, Museum Kunst Palast, Düsseldorf, Hayward Gallery, London, Centre Georges Pompidou, Paris and Mori Art Museum, Tokyo (2004–2005) and *Pattern Language: Clothing as Communicator*, University Art Museum, University of California, Santa Barbara (2006).

Reiko Sudo (b. Japan, 1953). Sudo's visionary combination of complex technologies, traditional techniques and new finishing processes has created extraordinary visual effects that have revolutionized textiles within interiors, fashion and art. Sudo founded the NUNO company in 1984 with Junichi Arai. Sudo's exhibitions include *2121: the Textile Vision of Reiko Sudo*, James Hockey Gallery, Farnham (2005).

Do-Ho Suh (b. South Korea, 1962). Suh received a BFA in painting from Rhode Island School of Design and an MFA in sculpture from Yale University. Many of his installations address the role of cloth in culture and the experience of cultural displacement. Suh has exhibited internationally for over a decade. He has held solo shows in Madrid and New York and at the Serpentine Gallery, London, and at the Fabric Workshop and Museum in Philadelphia.

Peter Testa. Testa is Principal in Charge of Design at Testa Architects based in Los Angeles. He was formerly a professor at MIT where he founded and directed the Emergent Design Group with students and faculty from Architecture, Engineering, Artificial Intelligence Lab and the Media Lab. His research and practice is internationally recognized for establishing a new design approach that synthesizes advances in engineering, material science and artificial intelligence to create a new organic minimalist architectural language. Testa has also held academic and research positions at Harvard University and Columbia University. He is the recipient of numerous awards including the Design Arts Award of the National Endowment for the Arts, the Graham Foundation Award and the MIT Innovation in Teaching Award.

Axel Thallemar (b. Germany, 1959). Trained as an engineer, Thallemer founded Festo AG and Co in 1994, transforming pneumatics manufacturing. Prior to this, he worked as a design engineer in the styling studio of Porsche, initiating the introduction of the computer-aided styling process. He has received numerous awards, especially for his Fluidic Muscle, which won Japan's Good

Design Award in 1998 and Germany's Federal Award for Product Design in 2000, among many others.

Manel Torres (b. Spain, 1974). Torres studied fashion design at undergraduate and postgraduate level before switching to the interrelated disciplines of design and science in his PhD supervised by the chemical engineering department at Imperial College, London. He worked as a designer for fashion houses in Japan, India and Europe, and designed his own range of jewelry and accessories. He has exhibited at London Fashion Week, the Crafts Council, the Science Museum, London, and in the United States and throughout Europe. Torres also acts as a consultant in various areas of the fashion and scientific industries. He has lectured internationally and his work has featured in numerous publications. He is currently the managing director of Fabrican Ltd and lectures at the Marangoni Institute in Milan on research and methodology.

Neils van Eijk (b. Netherlands, 1970) and Miriam van der Lubbe (b. Netherlands, 1972). Van Eijk and van der Lubbe share a playful, postmodern approach to design and work with familiar forms and traditional features of Dutch decorative art that they adapt and modify through the use of contemporary materials. They studied at the Design Academy Eindhoven and at the Sandberg Institute in Amsterdam and launched their own design studio in 1988. They work both collaboratively and separately and have exhibited at the European Ceramics Work Centre and the Textile Museum in Tilburg (2003) and in *Dutch at the Edge of Design* at the Museum of the Fashion Institute of Technology, New York (2005).

Roy Villevoye (b. Netherlands, 1960). Since the early 1990s Villevoye has worked in the Asmat Region of Papua New Guinea. His photographic work reflects the research-based ethnographic turn of contemporary art. *Rood Katoen (Red Calico)* was exhibited at the Rijksmuseum voor Volkenkunde in Leiden in 2001.

Auturo Vittori (b. Italy, 1971). Vittori studied architecture at the universities of Florence, Modena and Darmstadt. He set up his futuristic architectural practice Architecture and Vision in conjunction with Andreas Vogler in 2002. He has drawn upon the European Space Agency technology transfer programme for a number of his projects including *Desert Seal* which has recently been exhibited at the Museum of Modern Art in New York and at Futurotextiles in Lille.

Dré Wapenaar (b. Netherlands, 1961). Wapenaar has designed tents for a wide variety of activities, including camping, drinking coffee, selling flowers, reading newspapers, mass barbecues, for paying respects to the dead and for giving birth.

Marie Watt (born USA, 1960). Watt received an MA in painting and printmaking at Yale University School of Art. Since 2003 she has used blankets as a medium to explore a range of issues, including dreaming, cultural transmission and family history. Her work was exhibited in *Continuum: 12 Artists* (2003–2005) at the National Museum of the American Indian, Smithsonian Institution, New York. She currently teaches at Portland Community College.

Linda Worbin (b. Sweden, 1974). Worbin is a doctoral candidate at the Swedish School of Textiles at the University of Boras in Sweden researching the place of textile aesthetics in smart textiles. She previously worked at the Interactive Design Institute in Ivrea, Sweden, where she contributed textile designs to the IT+textiles Project.

Xuly Bët. Founded by Lamine Badian Kouyaté (b. Mali, 1962). Formerly trained as an architect in Paris, Kouyaté turned to fashion and launched his first collection in 1989. Working under his label Xuly Bët (which means 'watch out' in Wolof), Kouyaté has created an international fashion label from recycling multicultural local materials: the fabrics that he sources from the streets and flea markets surrounding his studio. He creates reknitted jumpers, dresses made of patchwork and painted T-shirts, and clothing made from African and Hawaiian prints overprinted with distinctive gold lettering. He was awarded the prestigious Creator of the Year award in 1994 by the *New York Times* and received the ANDAM awards in 1996. His label is sold all around the world.

Zephyr Technology. Launched by Brian Russell (New Zealand) in 2003, the company specializes in design and the supply of wearable smart fabrics. Zephyr design expertise includes pressure sensors integrated onto fabric (cloth, gadgets, surface), wireless transmission and integrated movement detectors (accelerometer, gyroscope). Zephyr is a privately owned New Zealand company established in 2003 and has recently secured private equity investment from iGLOBE Treasury to fund ongoing research and development.

Museums, Galleries and Design Institutes

AUSTRALIA

Faculty of Creative Arts
University of Wollongong
Northfields Avenue
Wollongong NSW 2522
The department of textiles has developed a specialized interest in cross-cultural textiles.

The Powerhouse Museum of Applied Arts
500 Harris Street Ultimo
Sydney NSW 1238
Australia's leading decorative arts and design museum, it houses an exceptional collection of contemporary textiles with a superbly annotated digital database.

AUSTRIA

Österreichisches Museum für Angewandte Kunst
Stubenring 5, 1010 Vienna

BELGIUM

Flanders Fashion Institute
Nationalestraat 28/2
2000 Antwerp
FFI is the knowledge centre for fashion in Flanders.

CANADA

Design Exchange, DX
234 Bay Street
PO Box 18, Toronto Dominion Centre
Toronto, Ontario M5K 1B2

Museum of Anthropology, University of British Columbia
6393 N.W. Marine Drive
Vancouver, B.C. V6T 1Z2
The museum is internationally respected for its collections, research, teaching, exhibitions and community connections. It has a closed collection of more than 5,000 ethnographic textiles.

National Gallery of Canada
380 Sussex Drive
Ottawa, Ontario K1N 9N4
National collection of art, including contemporary Native American work.

The Textile Museum of Canada, Contemporary Gallery
55 Centre Avenue
Toronto, Ontario M5G 2H5
The museum's permanent collection contains more than 12,000 textiles and spans almost 2,000 years and 200 world regions. It is dedicated to celebrating historic and contemporary textile expressions from around the world.

DENMARK

Danish Design Centre
27 Hans Christian Andersens Boulevard
1553 Copenhagen V
Distinguished by its experimental approach to exhibiting textiles, the centre's resources include an online database of designers.

Kunstindustrimuseet
(Danish Museum of Art and Design)
Bredgade 68, 1260 Copenhagen
Scandinavia's leading venue for exhibitions on industrial design and decorative art; houses a strong textiles collection.

FRANCE

Musée de la Mode et du Textile
Palais du Louvre
107 rue de Rivoli, 75001 Paris
The exhibition programme shows a marked emphasis on high fashion.

Musée de L'Impression sur Etoffes, Mulhouse
14 rue Jean-Jacques Henner
BP 1468–68072 Mulhouse
Outstanding collection of 18th- and 19th-century printed fabrics.

Musée des Tissus et des Arts Décoratifs
34 rue de la Charité
69002 Lyon
Outstanding collection of Lyonese silks and oriental fabrics.

Museum of Art and Industry
2 Place Louis Comte
42000 Saint Etienne
St Etienne was formerly the centre for jacquard ribbon weaving in France; the museum houses the world's largest collection of ribbons.

Saint Etienne International Design Biennale
Ecole des Beaux-Arts de St Etienne
15, rue Henri–Gonnard
42000 Saint-Etienne
Launched in 1998, the programme embraces food, design and fashion, and features work by designers from Morocco, Nigeria, Senegal, Japan, Europe and the Americas.

GERMANY

Deutsches Textilmuseum
(German Textile Museum)
Andreasmarkt 8, 47809 Krefeld
Houses a substantial international collection of textiles.

German Design Council (Rat für Formgebung)
PO Box 15 03 11, 60063 Frankfurt am Main
Mounts exhibitions, competitions and organizes a scheme of accreditation called the Red Dot Awards.

INDIA

Calico Museum of Textiles
Sarabhai Foundation Galleries
Shahibag, Ahmedabad, Gujarat
The textile collections are of exceptional historical value, comprising court textiles used by the Mughal and provincial rulers, trade textiles produced for export markets from the 15th to the 19th centuries, 19th-century regional embroideries, tie-dyed textiles and religious textiles.

Crafts Museum
Indian Institute of Art and Industry
17 Park Street, Kolkata

India Habitat Centre
Visual Arts Gallery
Lodhi Road, New Delhi 110003
Gallery, resource centre and conference facility promoting both the plastic and performing arts.

Indian Textile Museum
Marine Drive, South Mumbai

The Kutch Folk Art Museum of Textiles
Bhuj
Kutch 370001, Gujarat
Textiles and Indian nomadic embroidery.

The National Handcrafts and Handloom Museum
Pragati Maidan
Bhairon Road, 110001 New Delhi
Ikats, gold and silver brocades.

National Museum
Janpath 110011, New Delhi
Indian textiles and costumes (dating from the 17th to the 21st centuries), silks, ikats, rugs and painted fabrics.

ITALY

Galleria del Costume
1 Piazza Pitti, 50125 Florence
Dress, dating from the 18th century to the present day.

Museo del Tessuto
Via Santa Chiara 24, 59100 Prato
The collection features both historical and contemporary textiles.

JAPAN

Gallery Concept 21
3–15–16 Kita-aoyama
Minato-ku, 107–0061 Tokyo
Fashion-related exhibitions.

Gallery Ma
TOTO Nogizaka building 3F
1–24–3 Minami-aoyama, Minato-ku.
Tokyo 107–0062
Specializes in architecture and design; the gallery takes its name from the Japanese concept 'ma', which symbolically links humans, time and space.

The Kyoto Costume Institute
103 Shichijo
Goshonouchi Minamimachi
Kyoto 600–8864

Motoazabu Gallery
3–12–3 Motoazabu
Minato-ku, 106–0046 Tokyo

The National Museum of Modern Art, Kyoto
Okazaki Enshoji-cho
Sakyo-ku, Kyoto 606–8344

The National Museum of Modern Art, Crafts Gallery
3–1 Kitanomaru-koen
Chiyoda-ku, Tokyo 102–8322

Plus Minus Gallery
TEPCO Ginzakan 3F
6–11–1 Ginza
Chuo-ku, Tokyo 104–0061
Exhibits textile sculpture.

Senbikiya Gallery
1–1–9 Kyobashi
Chuoku 104–0031, Tokyo

Tokyo Textile Forum
2–18–1 Mathabura
Setagaya-ku, Tokyo
Teaching, exhibitions and magazine art forum.

MEXICO

Mexico Design Promotion Center
Avenue Insurgentes Sur 1855
Piso 10
Col. Guadalupe Inn, 01020 Mexico, D.F.

THE NETHERLANDS

Centraal Museum
Nicolaaskerkhof 10, Utrecht
The museum has a large and varied collection of art divided into five departments: old masters, modern art, design, fashion and local history.

Museum voor Volkenkunde Leiden (National Museum of Ethnology)
Steenstraat 1
Postbus 212, 2300 AE Leiden
Contemporary exhibitions plus permanent collections of objects from South-East Asia and the Pacific.

Nederlands Textielmuseum
Goirkestraat 96, 5046 GN Tilburg
Strong exhibition programme of both contemporary and historical textiles.

NEW ZEALAND

Auckland Art Gallery
Corner of Wellesley and Kitchener Streets
Auckland
Largest collection of contemporary art in New Zealand.

Museum of New Zealand Te Papa Tongarewa
Cable Street, Wellington
Features contemporary displays of Polynesian artefacts from Aotearoa and the Pacific Islands; a strong textile collection.

Tautai Contemporary Pacific Arts Trust
PO Box 68 339
Newton
Auckland
Promotes contemporary Pacific art and educates, mentors and supports both emerging and established artists.

NIGERIA

African Studies Gallery
University of Nigeria, Nsukka
University Road, Enugu

Asele Institute
Cultural centre and collection of contemporary African art housed in the house of Uche Okeke in Nimo.

The Junkyard Museum of Awkward Things
Lagos
Alternative art museum created by artist Dilomprizulike from rags and junk found on the streets.

NORWAY

Kunstindustrimuseet
St Olavs gate 1, Oslo
Houses a collection of Norwegian textiles dating from the 7th century to the present day.

POLAND

Central Museum of Textiles
282 Piotrkowska Street, 93–034 Lodz

SENEGAL
Biennale de l'Art Africain Contemporain
Biennale de Dakar
19, avenue Albert Sarraut
BP 3865 Dakar

SOUTH AFRICA
Design Institute South Africa
South African Bureau of Standards
1 Dr Lategan Road
Groenkloof, Pretoria 0001
Operates NAD (the online Network
of African Designers) and co-ordinates
the Design for development awards.

SWEDEN
Textilmuseet
Druveforsvägen 8, 504 33 Borås

SWITZERLAND
Musée Cantonal des Beaux Arts
Palais de Rumine
6 place de la Riponne
Lausanne CH 1014
Home to the Lausanne Biennale.

Textilmuseum
Vadianstrasse 2, St Gallen CH 9000

UK
Ashmolean Museum
Beaumont Street
Oxford OX1 2PH
The museum holds more than
4,000 textiles and is planning a
major new textiles gallery, which
will examine the place of textiles
in inter-Asian trade.

The British Museum
Great Russell Street
London WC1B 3DG
Holds a world-renowned collection
of textiles from Africa, the Pacific, the
Americas and Asia.

Constance Howard Resource and
Research Centre in Textiles
Goldsmiths College, University of London
Deptford Town Hall
New Cross Road, London SE14 6AF
Houses a growing collection of textile
art and other textiles used by teachers
at the Goldsmiths school of textiles.

Crafts Council Gallery
44a Pentonville Road, London N1 9BY
Promotes contemporary craft. Lively
contemporary exhibitions, including
knitting and textile recycling.

Design Museum
Shad Thames
London SE1 2YD

A museum of contemporary
international design. The website
features a superb online database
of designers.

Horniman Museum
100 London Road
Forest Hill
London SE23 3PQ
80, 000 ethnographic objects,
including a strong collection of textiles.

Ikon Gallery
1 Oozells Square
Brindley Place
Birmingham B1 2HS
One of the first galleries to recognize
the potential of fabric as a medium of
artistic exploration and has remained
a champion of experimental work.

The October Gallery
24 Old Gloucester Street
London WC1N 3AL
Founded in 1978, the October Gallery
is an art gallery dedicated to the
appreciation of art from all cultures
around the world. It has achieved
international recognition for its
exhibitions of work by contemporary
artists from West Africa and Papua
New Guinea.

Oriel Mostyn Art Gallery
12 Heol Vaughan
Llandudno LL30 1AB
Shows major international artists.

Pitt Rivers Museum
South Parks Road
Oxford OX1 3PP
Houses over half a million
archaeological and ethnographic
objects from all over the world.

Science Museum
Exhibition Road
London SW7 2DD
The Challenge of Materials Gallery
concentrates on man-made materials.

University of Cambridge University
Museum of Archaeology and
Anthropology
Dowing Street
Cambridge CB2 3DZ
50,000 ethnographic objects and
a lively exhibition programme.

Victoria and Albert Museum
Cromwell Road
London SW7 2RL
A world-renowned museum of
decorative art and design. The national

collection of textiles covers a period
of more than 2,000 years. It has a broad
geographic range with a particular
emphasis on Europe and India.

Whitworth Art Gallery
The University of Manchester
Oxford Road
Manchester M15 6ER
Renowned for its collection of Arts
and Craft textiles, the gallery also hosts
exhibitions of contemporary textiles.

UNITED STATES
Art in General
79 Walker Street
New York, NY 10013
An alternative art space with
exhibitions curated by artists. It also
maintains an artist-in-residence
program.

Artrain USA
1100 N. Main St.
Ste. 106, Ann Arbor, MI 48104
Artrain USA is an art museum housed
in vintage rail cars. It brings world-
class art exhibitions and art education
programs to communities and their
residents.

Bernice P. Bishop Museum
1525 Bernice Street
Honolulu, Hawaii, HI 96817
The museum has over 2.4 million
cultural artefacts representing the
transformation of native Hawaiian,
Pacific Island and immigrant
cultural life.

Brooklyn Museum
200 Eastern Parkway
New York, NY 11238–6052

Cooper-Hewitt, National Design
Museum (Smithsonian Institution)
2 East 91st Street
New York, NY 10128
The United States's pre-eminent
museum of design and decorative
art, it houses a world-renowned
collection of contemporary and
historical textiles including an
exceptional collection of samplers.

The Design Center at Philadelphia
University
Goldie Paley House
4200 Henry Avenue
Philadelphia, PA 19144–5497
Houses 200,000 Western and non-
Western textiles and costumes dating
from the 1st century AD to the present,
representing nearly every country in

the world, including an extraordinary
assembly of 19th- and early 20th-
century textiles, textile-related
artefacts and tools that document the
emergence of Philadelphia as one of the
United States's great textile producers
of the time. Also a critical resource for
research on American industrial design.

The Fabric Workshop and Museum
(FWM)
1315 Cherry Street
5th and 6th Floors
Philadelphia, PA 19107–2026
Founded in 1977, the FWM initially
offered artists the opportunity to explore
silkscreen printing on fabric. The
collection now has over 5,500 objects
created by more than 400 artists.

Museum at the Fashion Institute
of Technology
Seventh Avenue at 27th Street
New York, NY 10001–5992

MAD Museum of Arts and
Design New York
40 West 53rd Street, New York, NY 10019
Collects and exhibits contemporary
objects created in clay, glass, wood,
metal and fibre.

Museum of Craft and Folk Art San
Francisco
51 Yerba Buena Lane
San Francisco, CA 94103
Exhibits traditional and contemporary
folk art and craft from around the world.

Museum of Indian Arts and Culture
and the Laboratory of Anthropology
708 Camino Lejo, Santa Fe, NM 87504
Key collection of native art and
material culture; tells the stories of
the people of the Southwest from pre-
history through to contemporary art.

Museum of Modern Art (MOMA)
11 West 53 Street,
between Fifth and Sixth avenues
New York, NY 10019–5497
Note the design exhibition programme.

National Museum of African Art
(Smithsonian Institution)
950 Independence Ave, SW
Washington, DC 20560
Houses the primary collections of
African art and material culture in
the United States.

Peabody Essex Museum
East India Square
Salem, MA 01970–3783

A major Asian art museum, featuring
a superb collection of Asian export
art extant and 19th-century Asian
photography. It houses the oldest
collections of Native American and
Oceanic art in the United States.

The Studio Museum Harlem
144 West 125th Street
New York, NY 10027
One of the leading museums of
African-American art in the United
States. It also promotes work by
international artists of African descent.

Smithsonian National Museum
of the American Indian
Located on three different sites:

The George Gustav Heye Center
Alexander Hamilton
US Custom House
One Bowling Green
New York, NY 10004

Cultural Resources Center
4220 Silver Hill Road
Suitland, MD 20746

NMAI on the National Mall
Fourth Street and Independence Ave., S.W.
Washington, DC 20560
The museum is dedicated to the
preservation, study and exhibition
of the history and arts of Native
Americans.

Web Resources
Bionis Network: Promotes the idea that
biomimicry may hold the key to top
industrial sustainability.

Biopolymer.net: Knowledge centre
and consultancy with expertise in
biopolymers.

Core77: Aimed at the industrial design
community, Core77 publishes articles,
blogs, podcasts, discussion forums,
an extensive event calendar, job
listings, a database of design firms,
schools, vendors and services.

Designboom: Design ezine with
pieces on art, architecture, fashion,
photography and graphics.

Dexigner: Online information service
for designers and artists.

Doors of Perception: A conference,
online network and a weblog,
co-ordinated by John Thackara, which

harnesses some of the most innovative thinkers and practitioners to develop better solutions for sustainable design.

Honey Bee Network: Network for strengthening grassroots creativity. The Honeybee network covers over 77 countries. The online database includes innovations in textile manufacture and production filed by artisans and farmers.

Inhabitat: The blog and online magazine is updated daily to provide contemporary information on innovations in sustainable architecture and green design for the home.

Inneurotex: European platform for textile innovation.

Massive Change: Wide-ranging project on the nature and potential of design co-ordinated by Bruce Mau. To date, Massive Change has taken on the form of a travelling exhibition, a book, a series of formal and informal public events, a radio programme, an online forum and a blog. It takes a critical look at the current place of design (understood in the broadest sense of its economic, political, cultural and environmental impacts) and assesses what needs to be done in order to improve its outcomes.

Nextiles (Tex.in): A comprehensive online database for the textile and apparel industries.

Onsustain: An online platform to market sustainable design and designers by means of a showroom where products can be purchased; offers interviews with relevant designers.

TextileArts.net: Virtual arts centre developing web and community resources for artists, students, tutors, researchers and businesses involved in art textiles.

Transmaterial: Online catalogue and blog of innovative materials edited by architect Blaine E. Brownell.

Tree Hugger: American blog dedicated to green living.

Wearable Electronic and Smart Textiles Network (WEST): The WEST website is a space for industry and academia to find out about the latest developments in wearable electronic and smart textiles.

Worldchanging: A weblog of the most innovative solutions, ideas and inventions emerging today for building a sustainable future.

youthXchange: Developed by UNEP (United Nations Education Programme) and UNESCO (United Nations Educational, Scientific and Cultural Organisation), the website and book offers an educational resource devoted to the promotion of sustainable consumption.

Research Institutes

Autex, University of Ghent
Association for technical textile educational establishments run by Professor Paul Kiekens at the University of Ghent.

Centre for Alternative Technology,
Aberystwyth
Machynlleth
Powys SY20 9AZ

Centre for Biomimetics University of Reading
School of Construction Management and Engineering
Engineering Building
The University of Reading
Whiteknights
Reading RG6 6AY
Research into new materials and technologies inspired by nature.

The Centre for Sustainable Design
University College for the Creative Arts
Farnham Campus
Faculty of Design
Falkner Road
Farnham
Surrey GU9 7DS
Facilitates discussion and research on eco-design and environmental, economic, ethical and social considerations in product and service development and design. This is achieved through training and education, research, seminars, workshops, conferences, consultancy, publications and the Internet. The Centre also acts as an information clearing house and a focus for innovative thinking on sustainable products and services.

E Paggio research centre
University of Pisa

Lungarno Pacinotti
43–56126 Pisa
Specializes in kinesthetic sensing and smart fabrics.

Ecole Polytechnique Fédérale de Lausanne
Laboratoire de Technologie des Poudres
MX Ecublens
1015 Lausanne
Specialists in nano powders for textile coatings, photovoltaic fibres and wound dressings.

European Space Agency Technology Transfer Programme
PO Box 299
2200 AG Noordwijk
The Netherlands
European technology platform for the future of textiles and clothing.

Future Force Warrior
A US military initiative, part of the Future Combat Systems project, which envisions the radical use of technologies such as nanotechnology and magnetic fluid-based body armour, computer wearables and technologically enhanced textiles.

Heriott Watt University Research Institute for Flexible Materials
Scottish Borders Campus
Netherdale
Galashiels TD1 3HF

Hong Kong Polytechnic
QT715, The Institute of Textiles and Clothing
The Hong Kong Polytechnic University
Hunghom
Kowloon
Fashion design and textile technology innovation is one of the university's areas of strategic development.

Indian Institute of Technology
The Department of Textile Technology
Hauz Khas
New Delhi 110 016
Research institution involved in developing both active smart and very active smart (intelligent) textile materials for apparel or technical applications into aerospace, defence and sports.

Institute of Soldier Nanotechnologies at MIT
Building NE47, 4th Floor
77 Massachusetts Avenue
Cambridge, MA 02139

Intended to run between 2002 and 2007, the Institute of Soldier Nanotechnologies is a US Army-funded research initiative that aims to advance soldier survivability through advanced research into nanotechnology. It aims to develop a 21st-century battlesuit through the convergence of a number of discrete research programmes into the development of technology-rich textiles.

Intelligent Polymer Research Institute, University of Wollongong
Professor Gordon Wallace (Research Director)
ARC Centre of Excellence for Electromaterials Science
Intelligent Polymer Research Institute, University of Wollongong
Wollongong NSW 2522
Australia
Developed a world reputation for its research in the area of intelligent polymers.

Interactive Institute Göteborg Sweden
Box 1197
164 26 Kista
Sweden
The IT+textiles Project, Re-form Studio studies the use of textile aesthetics in computer interface, integration of computing within fabric and the use of smart materials to monitor energy flows.

Johnson Space Center
1601 Nasa Road
Houston, TX 77058
Led design projects such as Robonaut.

NASA (National Aeronautics and Space Administration)
The NASA Glenn Research Center Materials Division
21000 Brookpark Road
Cleveland, OH 44135
Research into superalloys, intermetallics and new fibres to be used in engine components for the space shuttle.

Natick Soldier Systems Center
Natick, Massachusetts
Responsible for researching, developing, fielding and managing food, clothing, shelters, airdrop systems and soldier support systems.

RIFleX Research Institute for Flexible Materials, Heriott Watt University
Scottish Borders Campus
Netherdale
Galashiels TD1 3HF

Research Institute for Flexible Materials based at the School of Textiles and Design of Heriot-Watt University.

Rocky Mountain Institute
1739 Snowmass Creek Road
Snowmass, CO 81654–9199
An NGO that aims to foster the efficient and restorative use of resources to make the world secure, just, prosperous and life-sustaining. They consult businesses, communities, individuals and governments about how to create more wealth and employment, protect and enhance natural and human capital, increase profit and competitive advantage, largely by doing what they do far more efficiently.

Tampere University Finland, Department of Computer Design. Wearable computers are a special example of mobile computers. They are either embedded in clothing, or they may even be the clothing. The aim in developing wearable computers is to provide the user with instant and easy-to-use access to digital information sources anytime, anywhere.

Winchester School of Art
University of Southampton
Textile Conservation Centre
Park Avenue
Winchester SO23 8DL
In an innovative collaborative venture, the Textile Conservation Centre, University of Southampton and the Victoria and Albert Museum, London, are seeking to develop sustainable solutions to the care and conservation of contemporary fabrics. Techno textiles and smart fabrics are at the cutting edge of technology developments. These textiles are entering museum collections as examples of fine art, haute couture and high-tech sportswear as well as innovative medical and industrial equipment.

Trade Fairs

Avantex Trade Fair for Innovative Textile Clothing, Frankfurt

Techtextil International Trade Fair for Technical Textiles and Non Wovens

WIRED NextFest, San Francisco, features innovations in communication, design, entertainment, exploration, health, transportation, security and green living.

Bibliography

General

Beattie, Alan, 'Follow the Thread', the *Financial Times*, 21 July 2006

Burn, Jonathan, Hilary Cottam, et al., *02 Transformation Design (Red Paper)*, London Design Council, 2006

Guidelines: A Handbook on the Environment for the Textile and Fashion Industry, The Sustainable Solution Design Association, Denmark, 2002

Kiekens, Paul, 'Textiles and Clothing in the Next Millennium: Quo Vadis?', online paper supplied by the Department of Engineering and Textiles, University of Ghent, 2005

Lutz, Walter, ed., *European Technology Platform for the Future of Textiles and Clothing, a Vision for 2020*, Euratex, 2004

Stylios, George, ed., *Interactive Smart Textiles: Innovation and Collaboration in Japan and South Korea*, Report of a Department of Trade and Industry Global Watch Mission, 2004

Thackara, John, *Putting the Future into Perspective*, Royal Society for the Encouragement of Arts, e-journal, June 2006

Wen, Geoffrey, *Globalization in Textiles. Corporate Stratergy and Competitive Advantage*, Pasold Lecture, London School of Economics, December 2001

Materials

Abouraddy, Ayman F., Jerimy Arnold, Mehmet Bayindir, Yoel Fink, John D. Joannopulous, 'Array Detectors: Fabrics that "See" Photosensitive Fibre Constructs' in *Optics and Photonics News*, issue no. 21, December 2006

Bayindir, Mehmet, et al., 'Metal-Insulator Semi-Conductor Optoelectronic Fibres' in *Nature*, 431, pp. 826–29, 2004

Benyus, Janine, *Biomimicry: Innovation Inspired by Nature*, New York, 1998

Bonser, Richard, 'Biomimetics' in *Biological Sciences Review*, April 2005

Brownell, Blaine E., *Transmaterial: A Catalog of Materials that Redefine our Physical Environment*, New York, 2006

Elices, Manuel, José Pérez-Rigueiro, Gustavo R. Plaza and Gustavo V. Guinea, 'Finding Inspiration in Argiope Trifasciata Spider Silk Fibers' in *The Journal of the Minerals, Metals and Materials Society*, February 2005

Hawken, Paul, et al., *Natural Capitalism: Creating the Next Industrial Revolution*, Boston, 2000

'Interactive Textiles: New Materials in the New Millennium' in *Journal of Industrial Textiles*, vol. 29, no. 3, January 2000

Jeronimidis, George, 'Electro-active Polymers', Smart Textiles Network (on-line resource)

Johnson, Brent, 'MIT Investigates Photonic Uniforms', Photonics.com, March 2003

Küchler, Susanne, 'Rethinking Textile: the Advent of the Smart Fiber Surface' in *Textile: the Journal of Cloth and Culture*, vol. 1, issue no. 3

Lawrence, C. and M. C. J. Large, 'Optical Biomimetics' in *Photonics Science News*, vol. 6, issue 1–2, pp. 6–21

Lendlein, Andreas, 'Shape Memory Polymers: Biodegradeable Sutures' in *Materials World*, vol. 10., no. 7, pp. 29–30, July 2002

Luzinov, Igor, et al., 'Ultrahydrophobic Fibers: Lotus Approach', *National Textile Center Annual Report*, 2005

McDonough, William, and Michael Braungart, 'The Promise of Nylon 6-BASF' in *Green@Work*, January–February 2002

McDonough, William, and Michael Braungart, 'Transforming the Textile Industry: Victor Innovatex' in *Green@Work*, June 2002

McDonough, William, and Michael Braungart, *Cradle to Cradle: Remaking the Way We Make Things*, New York, 2002

Motornov, M., S. Minko, K.- J. Eichhorn, M. Nitschke, F. Simon, M. Stamm, 'Reversible Tuning of Wetting Behavior of Polymer Surface with Responsive Polymer Brushes' in *Langmuir*, 19 (19), pp. 8077–8085, 2003

Newman, Cathy, 'Dreamweavers' in *National Geographic Magazine*, January 2003

Quinn, Bradley, *Techno Fashion*, Oxford, 2002

Thackara, John, *In the Bubble: Designing in a Complex World*, London and Cambridge, Mass., 2005

'Threads that Think', the *Economist*, 8 December 2005

Venema, Liesbeth, 'Optical Fibers, A light Fabric' in *Nature*, 431, 2004, p. 749

Vollrath, F., and D. P. Knight, 'Liquid Crystalline Spinning of Spider Silk' in *Nature*, 410, 2001, pp. 541–48

Wilton, Pete, 'The Wonder Stuff' in *Spotlight: Future Technologies (EPSRC)*, Spring 2005, pp. 20–23

Xiaoming Tao, ed., *Smart Fibres, Fabrics and Clothing*, Cambridge, 2001

Xiaoming Tao, ed., *Wearable Electronics and Photonics*, Cambridge and Boca Raton, Florida, 2005

Objects

Balmond, Cecil, and Jannuzzi Smith, *Informal*, Munich and London, 2002

Balmond, Cecil, et al., 'Engineering Marsyas at Tate Modern' in *The Arup Journal*, January 2003

Garcia, Mark (ed.), *Architextiles, Architectural Design*, London, 2006

Hemmings, Jessica, 'A Soft Touch: Interview with Maggie Orth' in *Selvedge Magazine*, November–December 2005

Hensel, Michael, Achim Menges, Michael Weinstock, *Techniques and Technologies in Morphogenetic Design (Architectural Design)*, London, 2006

Mazé, Ramia, Johan Redström and Maria Redström, *IT+Textiles*, Finland, 2005

Orth, M., R. Post, and E. B. Cooper, *Fabric Computing Interfaces Proceedings of Conference on Human Factors in Computing Systems (short paper)*, CHI '98 conference, Los Angeles, 1998

Testa, Peter, and Dervyn Weiser, 'Emergent Structural Morphology' in *Contemporary Techniques in Architecture*, London, 2004

Wigley, Mark, *White Walls, Designer Dresses: the Fashioning of Modern Architecture*, Cambridge, Mass. and London, 1995

Wiltshire, Alex, 'Tord Boontje' in *Icon*, July–August 2004

Pattern

Ball, Philip, *The Self Made Tapestry: Pattern Formation in Nature*, Oxford, 1999

Danet, Brenda, 'Pixel Patchwork: Quilting in Time on Line' in *Textile: the Journal of Cloth and Culture*, vol. 1, issue 2, 2003

Decorattivo 1, Milan, 1976

Decorattivo 2, Milan, 1977

Hoyle, Rebecca B., *Pattern Formation: An Introduction to Methods*, Cambridge, 2006

Jackson, Leslie, 'Eley Kishimoto: Fashion's Reluctant Stars' in *Icon*, September 2004

McCollough, M., *Abstracting Craft: the Practiced Digital Hand*, Cambridge, Mass. and London, 1996

Miller Daniel, and Don Slater, *The Internet: an Ethnographic Approach*, Oxford, 2001

Scheinman, Pamela, 'Linda Hutchins: Reiterations' in *American Craft*, vol. 64, no. 4, 2004

Textiles, Art and Culture

'African Fashion' in *Revue Noire Magazine*, no. 26, 1998

Anatsui, El, 'Sankofa: "Go back an' Pick", Three Studio Notes and a Conversation' in *Third Text*, 23, 1993

Bamgboyé, O. A. et al., *Writings on Technology and Culture*, Rotterdam, 2001

Becker, Carol, 'Amazwi Abesifazane' in *Art Journal* (College Art Association, New York), Winter 2004

Bolton, Lissant, *Unfolding the Moon: Enacting Women's Kastom in Vanuatu*, Honolulu, 2003

Brunel, Charlotte, *The T-shirt Book*, London and New York, 2002

Colchester, Chloë, *Clothing the Pacific*, Oxford, 2003

Hakem, Tewfik, 'Double Culture: Xuly Bët, Lamine Badian Kouyaté', FranceCulture.com (transcription of a radio interview), 4 January 2005

Herbst, Toby, and Joel Kopp, *The Flag in American Indian Art*, New York, 1993

Hoggart, Liz, 'Grayson Perry: the Heraldry of the Subconscious' in *Selvedge*, issue 00 (launch issue), May 2004

Lewis-Harris, Jacquelyn A., 'Not Without a Cost: Contemporary PNG Art in the 21st Century' in *Visual Anthropology*, vol. 17, no. 3–4, July–December 2004

Oguibe, Olu, 'Beyond Death and Nothingness' in *African Arts*, vol. 31, no. 1, 1998

Oguibe, Olu, 'El Anatsui in the Public Place', *Third Text*, Issue 23, Summer 1993

Oguibe, Olu, and Salah M. Hassan, *Authentic/Ex-centric: Conceptualism in Contemporary African Art*, New York, 2001

Picton, J., 'Undressing Ethnicity: the Art of Yinka Shonibare' in *African Arts*, Autumn 2001

Pinto, Robert, Nicolas Bourriaud and Maia Damianovic, *Lucy Orta*, London, 2003

Rowley, Sue, *Reinventing Textiles. Volume 1: Tradition and Innovation*, Exeter, 1999

Sharrad, Paul, and Anne Collett, *Reinventing Textiles. Volume 3: Postcolonialism and Creativity*, Exeter, 2001

Exhibition Catalogues

Antonelli, Paola, *Safe: Design Takes on Risk*, New York: Museum of Modern Art, 2005

Brand, J., and J. Teunissen, *Global Fashion Local Tradition: On the Globalisation of Fashion*, Utrecht: Utrecht Centraal Museum, 2005–2006

Double Dress, Jerusalem: The Israel Museum, 2002

El Anatsui: Gawu, Llandudno: Oriel Mostyn Gallery, Wales, 2003

Fabrics of Change: Trading Identities, University of Wollongong, 2004

Futurotextiles, Lille, 2006–2007

Import Export: Global Influences in Contemporary Design, London: Victoria and Albert Museum, 2005

Kibung: Textiles from the Graduates of the National Arts School, Papua New Guinea, Brisbane: The University of Queensland, 2003

Kitsch Kitsch Hota Hai, New Delhi: Gallery Espace, India Habitat Centre, 2001

Knit 2 Together: Concepts and Knitting, London: The Crafts Council, 2006

Leonard, Polly, and Janice Jeffries, *Boys Who Sew*, London: The Crafts Council, 2003

McQuaid, Matilda, *Extreme Textiles: Designing for High Performance*, New York: Cooper-Hewitt, National Design Museum, Smithsonian Institution, 2005

Njami, Simon (ed.), *Africa Remix: Contemporary Art of a Continent*, London: Hayward Gallery, 2005

O'Neill, Ani, *Cottage Industry*, Wellington: City Gallery, 1997

Pasifika Styles, Museum of Anthropology and Archaeology, Cambridge, 2006

Picton, J., *The Art of African Textiles: Technology, Tradition and Lurex*, London: Barbican Art Gallery, 1995

Static!, Chicago: Wired Next Fest, 2005

Uncomfortable Truths: the Shadow of the Slave Trade in Art and Design, London: Victoria and Albert Museum, 2007

Villevoye, Roy, *Rood Katoen (Red Calico)*, Leiden: Rijksmuseum voor Volkenkunde, 2001

Watt, Marie, *Blanket Stories: Receiving*, Portland, Oregon: Ronna and Eric Hoffmann Gallery of Contemporary Art, 2005

Well Fashioned: Eco Style in the UK, London: The Crafts Council, 2006–2007

Who Stole the Tee Pee?, New York: National Museum of the American Indian, Smithsonian Institution, 2001

Yinka Shonibare: Double Dutch, Rotterdam: Museum Boijmans van Beuningen, 2004

Glossary

actuators Textile actuators or muscles are the active components of smart fibres. They are currently made from polymer gels and membranes.

aramids Strong synthetic fibres with good heat resistance; renown for their use in bullet-proof vests or for ballistic protection. Initially developed in the mid-1960s, aramid fibres are produced from spinning a fibre from a liquid chemical blend. Kevlar (DuPont), for example, requires the use of concentrated sulphuric acid in its manufacture in order to keep the highly insoluble polymeric solution soluble during the process of synthesis and spinning.

barkcloth (tapa) Fabric typically made from the beaten inner bark of the paper mulberry tree; used traditionally in the Pacific Islands and by other Austronesian speaking peoples.

biological nutrient A biodegradable product that promotes the health of the natural environment.

biomimicry In the strictest definition of the term, biomimicry denotes design based upon the mimesis not merely of natural forms and natural materials, but of the economy of natural ecological systems.

biopolymer A polymer generated from a renewable natural resource; can be made with plants, animals or micro organisms or they can be chemically synthesized from materials such as corn starch, seaweed, oil, etc. They are an alternative to petroleum-based plastics.

bluetooth technology An industrial specification for wireless communication networks.

carbon fibre Refers to a carbon filament or thread and, by extension, to a cloth made from this material. Carbon fibre is made by baking fibres made from other materials such as rayon, polyacrylonitrile or pitch in an inert, oxygen-free oven.

carbon nanotube Thin tubes of carbon atoms that are one nanometre in diameter and have extraordinary properties in terms of their strength, conductivity and flexibility. When they were discovered by in the mid-1990s they were heralded as the miracle fibre of the 21st century, a replacement for silicon (which is inflexible) in integrated circuits, and it was thought they would bring about a new era of flexible electronics. However so far they have proved difficult to manufacture in industrial quantities.

closed-loop manufacture A model of manufacture that mimics the natural behaviour of living plants which recycle their materials without generating net waste. It is contrasted with the linear pattern of production: mine, use, dipose that was developed before pressure upon natural resources became an issue.

conductive yarns Most of the commercially available conductive and semi-conductive yarns are composite materials made from non-conductive polymers containing conductive metallic wires, particles, powders or coatings that adversely affect the flexibility and washability of products that are made from them. Research is currently under way to produce inherently conductive polymers that are created by doping, i.e., adding impurities (atoms) of another material in an inert environment.

dielectric mirror A special kind of a mirror made of a substrate of glass, or a polymeric material on which one or more thin layers of dielectric material are deposited to form an optical coating. By careful choice of the type and thickness of the dielectric layers, the range of wave lengths and amount of light reflected from the mirror can be specified. They have recently been produced in fibre form.

electroactive polymers *see* polymer gels

fairtrade An independent labelling scheme that was initially developed in the Netherlands in the 1980s and which is now in use in more than 20 different countries. Initially applied to food, its use has now been extended to textiles such as cotton. To qualify for use of the fairtrade label, traders must prove that they pay farmers a premium above the market value of their commodity which ensures that people can earn a sustainable living from farming and invest in suitable development schemes.

geotextiles Technical textiles used to control soil erosion.

hydrophilic and hydrophobic fibres and membranes Water absorbant and water repellant properties.

modular design Typically composed of smaller parts (modules) that can be assembled together in different ways.

nanotechnology The creation of functional materials and devices through the control of matter on the nanometre (i.e., a billionth of metre) scale.

optical fibre Made from glass or plastic and designed to guide light along its core by total internal reflection.

organic light emitting diodes (OLEDs) Illuminated solely by the movement of electrons in a semi-conducting material. They are self luminous and do not require any of the back lighting, diffusers or other items associated with liquid crystal displays. They are far more efficient than conventional incandescent bulbs and have potential use in flexible light-emitting textiles in the future. Recently scientists at Princeton and the University of Southern California have developed OLEDs on thin sheets of transparent plastic that are capable of mimicking natural light.

pattern formation Spontaneous pattern formation in non-linear distributed systems is regarded as a prime example of the emergent behaviour of complex systems.

photonic fibres Fibres that generate, detect, transmit or modulate photons (particles of light).

photovoltaic fibres As the name implies, photovoltaic cells convert sunlight (photo) into electricity (voltaic). PV cells have conventionally been made from semi-conductive materials such as silicon. PV films developed in the late 1990s were less efficient, but far more user friendly. Research is now advanced into the development of PV fibres.

polymer The term polymer is derived from the Greek words *polys* meaning many and *meros* meaning parts. A key feature that distinguishes polymers from other molecules is that they are composed of many identical or complementary sub-units, monomers that are linked together. Synthetic polymer fibres were first produced in the mid-1930s.

polymer gels Consist of a polymer network that is inflated with a solvent such as water. They have the ability to swell up or shrink in response to external stimuli such as an electric current.

preform A piece of material used to draw an optical fibre.

quotas From 1974 until 1995 global textile trade was governed by the Multifibre Arrangement (MFA). This was a framework of bilateral agreements (i.e., specific trade deals between two countries) and unilateral trade agreements that limited the quantities of specific categories of textile goods that could be imported by the ageing industrial economies. After a decade of adjustment, quotas were to have been definitively lifted in 2005, but a limited number of quoats have been reimposed as a temporary measure.

shape memory materials Materials that can memorize a permanent shape. They will return to this shape in response to an external stimulus such as heat or sunlight. Shape memory effects have been reported for different materials such as metallic alloys, ceramics, glasses, gels and polymers.

smart textiles Sense and respond to external stimuli from mechanical, thermal, chemical, electrical, magnetic or other sources. Passive smart materials sense environmental stimuli; active smart materials react to these conditions or stimuli; intelligent materials respond to stimuli in a pre-programmed fashion.

sustainable design An approach to design that seeks to ensure that the product improves the social and ecological environment.

tariffs Import duties used to increase the price of cheap imports.

technical nutrient A product that can be recycled into a secondary product of either comparable or improved quality.

textile scaffolds Increasingly used in tissue engineering. They have to be tailored for the specific use required.

tivaevae Appliquéd and patchworked cloths made in the Cook Islands, Niue and Tonga.

Photographic credits